PORTAL HYPERTENSION – CAUSES AND COMPLICATIONS

Edited by **Dmitry V. Garbuzenko**

Portal Hypertension – Causes and Complications
Edited by Dmitry V. Garbuzenko

Published by InTech

Janeza Trdine 9, 51000 Rijeka, Croatia

Publishing Process Manager Sandra Bakic

Technical Editor Teodora Smiljanic

Cover Designer InTech Design Team

Additional hard copies can be obtained from orders@intechopen.com

Portal Hypertension – Causes and Complications, Edited by Dmitry V. Garbuzenko
p. cm.
ISBN 978-953-51-0251-9

For EU product safety concerns:
IN TECH d.o.o., Prolaz Marije Krucifikse Kozulić 3, 51000 Rijeka, Croatia,
info@intechopen.com or visit our website at intechopen.com.

Meet the editor

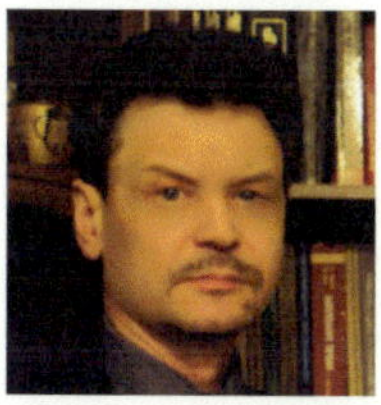

Prof. Dmitry V. Garbuzenko, MD was born in 1962 in Russia. In 1985 he graduated from Chelyabinsk State Medical Academy. From 1985 until 1990 he was the post-graduate student in Department of Hospital Surgery, ChSMA. Since 1990, Dr. Garbuzenko has been working in the Chelyabinsk State Medical Academy as professor in Department of Faculty Surgery. His scientific interests are problems connected with portal hypertension in patients with liver cirrhosis and study of pathophysiologic basis for its treatment. Dr. Garbuzenko is a member of Russian Gastroenterological Association and of International Association of Surgeons-Hepatologists. He has authored more than 100 publications, and has 2 inventions and 1 monograph ("Gastroesophageal variceal hemorrhage in cirrhotic patients: pathogenesis, prophylactic, treatment").

Contents

Preface

Portal hypertension is a clinical syndrome defined by a portal venous pressure gradient exceeding 5 mm Hg. It is initiated by increased outflow resistance, and can occur at a presinusoidal (intra- or extrahepatic), sinusoidal, or postsinusoidal level. As the condition progresses, there is a rise in portal blood flow, a combination that mains and worsens the portal hypertension.

Cirrhosis is the most common cause of portal hypertension in the Western world. There are more rare intrahepatic causes of portal hypertension, such as cystic fibrosis liver disease. Extra hepatic portal venous obstruction is found mainly at children, and it can also be caused by myeloproliferative diseases.

In cirrhosis, the principal site of increased resistance to outflow of portal venous blood is within the liver itself. Mesenteric arterial vasodilation is hallmark of cirrhosis and contributes to both increased portal venous inflow and a systemic hyperdinamic circulatory state. Arterial vasodilatation is regulated by a complex interplay of various vasodilator molecules and factors that influence the production of those vasodilator molecules.

Portal hypertension is associated with severe complications, including ascites, hepatic encephalopathy, hypersplenism, bleeding from gastro-esophageal varices. Despite the progress achieved over last decades, the 6-week mortality associated with variceal bleeding is still in the order of 10-20%. Endoscopic assessment of esophageal varices and the state of esophageal and stomach mucosa at the esophagogastroduodenoscopy, presents high importance for the assessment of risk of their development. However, invasiveness as well as discomfort that are tolerated by patients during the given procedure, lead to the rejection from it and therefore they can't be subjected to examination in a number of cases. Beside that, the research might be impossible to carry out in case if the state of patient is grave. The investigation of hepatic venous pressure gradient, that reflects the portal hypertension intensity best of all, haven`t been realized in the clinical practice up to now. Considering the above mentioned disadvantages of main methods, the development of additional prognostic criteria of the risk of esophageal varices bleeding remains the urgent problem of the internal medicine.

Current methods of treatments in portal hypertension include farmacologic therapy by vasoactive drugs, endoscopic therapy, portosystemic shunt surgery and transjugular intrahepatic portosystemic shunts (TIPS). Expansion in the knowledge of pathophysiology of portal hypertension is need as this might provide new and useful strategies for the future. The described problems above associated mainly with portal hypertension are presented in this book.

Dmitry V. Garbuzenko
Department of Surgical Diseases and Urology,
Chelyabinsk State Medical Academy, Chelyabinsk,
Russia

1

The Molecules: Abnormal Vasculatures in the Splanchnic and Systemic Circulation in Portal Hypertension

Yasuko Iwakiri
Yale University School of Medicine, USA

1. Introduction

Portal hypertension, defined as an increase in pressure within the portal vein, is a detrimental complication in liver diseases. The increased intrahepatic resistance as a consequence of cirrhosis is the primary cause of portal hypertension (Figure 1). Once it is developed, portal hypertension influences extrahepatic vascular beds in the splanchnic and systemic circulation. Two major consequences of portal hypertension in this regard are excessive arterial vasodilation/hypocontractility and the formation of portosystemic collateral vessels. Both excessive arterial vasodilation and portosystemic collateral vessel formation help to increase the blood flow through the portal vein and worsen portal hypertension. This facilitates the development of the abnormal hemodynamic condition, called the hyperdynamic circulatory syndrome, and ultimately leads to variceal bleeding and ascites (Bosch 2000; Bosch 2007; Groszmann 1993; Iwakiri 2011; Iwakiri & Groszmann 2006).

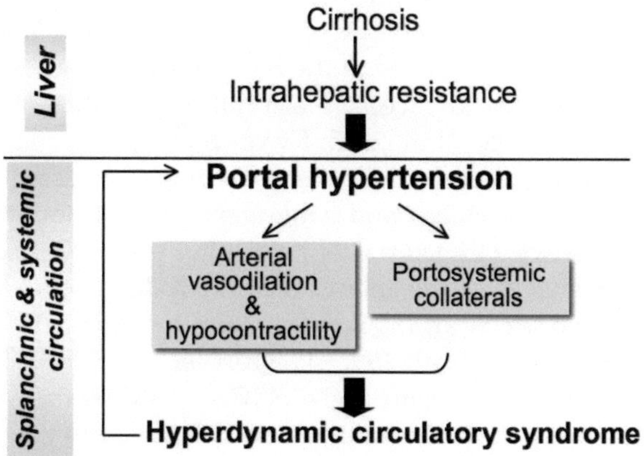

Fig. 1. Overview of portal hypertension.

This chapter summarizes current knowledge of molecules and factors that play critical roles in the development and maintenance of excessive arterial vasodilation and portosystemic collateral vessels in the splanchnic and systemic circulation in cirrhosis and portal hypertension. The chapter concludes with a brief discussion about the future directions of this area of study.

2. Key molecules and factors – Excessive arterial vasodilation/hypocontractility

This section addresses molecules and factors that are involved in the development and maintenance of excessive arterial vasodilation/hypocontractility in cirrhosis and portal hypertension.

2.1 Key molecules

The molecules discussed here include nitric oxide (NO), carbon monoxide (CO), prostacyclin (PGI_2), endocannabinoids, Endothelium-derived hyperpolarizing factor (EDHF), adrenomedullin, tumor necrotic factor alpha (TNFα), bradykinin and urotensin II. In addition to these vasodilatory molecules, decreased response to vasoconstrictors, such as neuropeptide Y, also contributes to hypocontractility of mesenteric arterial beds (i.e., arteries of the splanchnic circulation).

2.1.1 Nitric oxide

Nitric oxide (NO) is the most potent vasodilatory molecule in vessels and contributes to excessive arterial vasodilation in the splanchnic and systemic circulation in portal hypertension perhaps to the most significant degree. NO, synthesized by endothelial NO synthase (eNOS) in the endothelium, defuses into smooth muscle cells and activates guanylate cyclase (GC) to produce cyclic guanosine monophosphate (cGMP) (Arnold, et al. 1977; Furchgott & Zawadzki 1980; Ignarro, et al. 1987), facilitating vessel relaxation.

In portal hypertension, elevated eNOS activity causes overproduction of NO and the resultant excessive arterial vasodilation in the splanchnic and systemic circulation. As for the other two NOS isoforms, neuronal NOS (nNOS) and inducible NOS (iNOS), a couple of studies suggest that nNOS, which resides in the nerve terminus and smooth muscle cells of the vasculature, also contributes to excessive arterial vasodilation in portal hypertension, although its effect is small (Jurzik, et al. 2005; Kwon 2004). In contrast to eNOS and nNOS, which are constitutively expressed, iNOS is generally expressed in the presence of endotoxin and inflammatory cytokines and generates a large amount of NO. Interestingly, however, despite the presence of bacterial translocation and endotoxin in cirrhosis, iNOS has not been detected in arteries of the splanchnic and systemic circulation in cirrhosis and portal hypertension (Fernandez, et al. 1995; Heinemann & Stauber 1995; Iwakiri, et al. 2002; Morales-Ruiz, et al. 1996; Sogni, et al. 1997; Weigert, et al. 1995; Wiest, et al. 1999). This paradox remains to be elucidated. Accordingly, eNOS would be the most important among the three isoforms of NOS for excessive vasodilation observed in arteries of the splanchnic and systemic circulation in portal hypertension (Iwakiri 2011; Iwakiri & Groszmann 2006; Wiest & Groszmann 1999).

eNOS is regulated by complex protein-protein interactions, posttranslational modifications and cofactors (Sessa 2004). A summary of mechanisms that activate eNOS is shown in Figure 2. Below presented are several proteins that have been reported to increase eNOS activity in the superior mesenteric artery (i.e., an artery of the splanchnic circulation) of portal hypertensive rats.

2.1.1.1 Heat shock protein 90 (Hsp90)

This figure shows a general idea of eNOS regulation, not limited to portal hypertension. Caveolin-1 inhibits eNOS activity, while eNOS is activated through interactions with heat shock protein 90 (Hsp90), tetrahydrobiopterin (BH_4), guanosine triphosphate (GPT) and calcium calmodulin (CaM). Additionally, eNOS is phosphorylated and activated by Akt, also known as protein kinase B. VEGF; vascular endothelial growth factor, TNFα; tumor necrosis factor alpha.

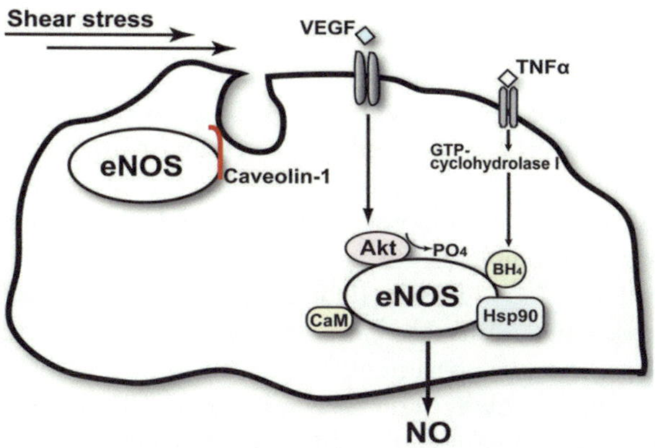

Fig. 2. Endothelial nitric oxide synthase (eNOS) is regulated by complex protein-protein interactions and posttranslational modifications.

A molecular chaperone, Hsp90, acts as a mediator of a signaling cascade leading to eNOS activation (Garcia-Cardena, et al. 1998). In the superior mesenteric artery isolated from portal hypertensive rats, an Hsp90 inhibitor, geldanamycin (GA), partially attenuated excessive vasodilation (Shah, et al. 1999). This observation suggests that Hsp90, at least in part, plays a role in elevated activation of eNOS, which causes overproduction of NO in the superior mesenteric artery in portal hypertensive rats.

2.1.1.2 Tetrahydrobiopterin (BH4)

eNOS requires BH_4 for its activity (Cosentino & Katusic 1995; Mayer & Werner 1995). Cirrhosis increases circulating endotoxin, which elevates activity of guanosine triphosphate (GPT)-cyclohydrolase I, an enzyme that generates BH_4. One study shows that increased levels of BH_4, as a result of cirrhosis, enhance eNOS activity in the superior mesenteric artery (Wiest, et al. 2003). Thus, an increase in BH_4 production in the superior mesenteric artery of cirrhotic rats is thought to be one of the mechanisms by which eNOS contributes to excessive arterial vasodilation.

2.1.1.3 Akt/protein kinase B

Akt, a serine/threonine kinase, can directly phosphorylate eNOS on Serine1177 (human) or Serine1179 (bovine) and activates eNOS, leading to NO production (Dimmeler, et al. 1999; Fulton, et al. 1999). We have shown that portal hypertension increases eNOS phosphorylation by Akt in the superior mesenteric artery and that wortmannin, an inhibitor of the phosphatidylinositol-3-OH-kinase (PI3K)/Akt pathway, decreases NO production and excessive vasodilation in the superior mesenteric artery isolated from portal hypertensive rats (Iwakiri, et al. 2002). These observations suggest that Akt-dependent phosphorylation and activation of eNOS play a role in excessive NO production and the resulting vasodilation in the superior mesenteric artery of portal hypertensive rats.

Since eNOS is the major NOS that generates NO in arteries of the splanchnic and systemic circulation, understanding the mechanisms by which eNOS is activated in these arteries is essential and allows us to develop critical strategies to block excessive arterial vasodilation and the subsequent development of the hyperdynamic circulatory syndrome.

2.1.2 Carbon monoxide (CO)

CO is an end product of the heme oxygenase (HO) pathway and a potent vasodilatory molecule that functions in a similar mechanism to NO (Figure 3). It activates sGC in vascular smooth muscle cells and regulates the blood flow and resistance in several vascular beds (Naik & Walker 2003). HO has two isoforms, HO-1 and HO-2. HO-1, also known as heat shock protein 32, is an inducible isoform. HO-2, a ubiquitously expressed constitutive isoform, is also found in blood vessels (Ishizuka, et al. 1997; Zakhary, et al. 1996). In pathological conditions, HO activity increases markedly due to the up-regulation of HO-1 (Cruse & Lewis 1988). Several experimental and clinical studies have shown a possible relationship between HO pathway and several complications of cirrhosis and portal hypertension, such as cardiac dysfunction (Liu, et al. 2001), renal dysfunction (Miyazono, et al. 2002), hepatopulmonary syndrome (Carter, et al. 2002), spontaneous bacterial peritonitis (De las Heras, et al. 2003) and viral hepatitis (Tarquini, et al. 2009).

Increased portal pressure alone contributes to the activation of HO pathway in mesenteric arteries and other organs (Angermayr, et al. 2006; Fernandez & Bonkovsky 1999). In a study using rats with partial portal vein ligation, a surgical model that induces portal hypertension, HO-1 was up-regulated in the superior mesenteric arterial beds (Angermayr, et al. 2006). When rats with partial portal vein ligation were given an HO inhibitor, tin(Sn)-mesoporphyrin IX, intraperitoneally immediately after surgery for the following 7 days, a significant reduction in portal pressure was observed in the HO inhibitor-treated group compared to the placebo group. However, the HO inhibition did not affect the formation of portosystemic collaterals in portal hypertensive rats (Angermayr, et al. 2006).

Like those surgically induced portal hypertensive rats, rats with cirrhosis exhibit enhanced HO pathway to mediate excessive vasodilation in arteries of the splanchnic and systemic circulation (Chen, et al. 2004; Tarquini, et al. 2009). Rats with bile duct ligation (a surgical model of biliary cirrhosis) showed an increase in HO-1 expression in both the superior mesenteric artery and the aorta, compared to sham-operated rats. In contrast, HO-2 expression did not differ between the two groups of rats. Importantly, aortic HO activities as well as blood CO levels were positively related to the degree of the hyperdynamic circulatory syndrome assessed by mean arterial pressure, cardiac input and peripheral vascular resistance. Acute administration of an HO inhibitor, zinc protoporphyrin (ZnPP), ameliorated the hyperdynamic circulatory syndrome in cirrhotic rats with 4 weeks after bile duct ligation (Chen, et al. 2004; Tarquini, et al. 2009).

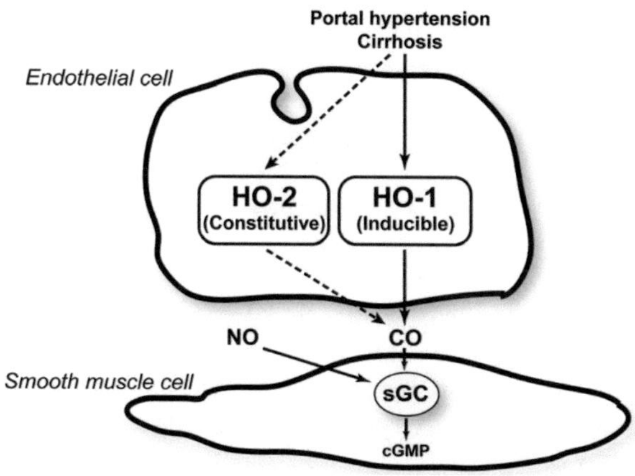

Fig. 3. Hemeoxygenase (OH) pathway in the arterial splanchnic and systemic circulation in cirrhosis and portal hypertension. HO-1 is an inducible isoform, while HO-2 is a constitutive isoform. Both nitric oxide (NO) and carbon monoxide (CO) activate soluble guanylate cyclase (sGC) in smooth muscle cells and facilitate vasodilation.

In contrast to other studies, a study by Sacerdoti et al. (Sacerdoti, et al. 2004) reported that HO-2, not the inducible HO-1, was up-regulated in mesenteric arteries of cirrhotic rats. In their study, cirrhotic rats were generated by giving carbon tetrachloride (CCl_4) in gavage for 8 to 10 weeks. Consistent with other studies, however, administration of an HO inhibitor, tin(Sn)-mesoporphyrin IX, ameliorated excessive arterial vasodilation in cirrhotic rats. Collectively, these observations may suggest that different experimental models of cirrhosis and portal hypertension cause different effects on HO pathway in the aorta and mesenteric arteries, thus resulting in up-regulation of different types of HO isoforms.

Studies with cirrhotic patients also showed an increase in plasma CO levels (De las Heras, et al. 2003; Tarquini, et al. 2009). Spontaneous bacterial peritonitis further accelerated blood CO levels in cirrhotic patients (De las Heras, et al. 2003). Furthermore, Tarquini et al. (Tarquini, et al. 2009) documented that plasma CO levels as well as HO expression and activity in polymorphonuclear cells were significantly increased in patients with viral hepatitis and the hyperdynamic circulatory syndrome. Importantly, plasma CO levels were directly correlated with the severity of the hyperdynamic circulatory syndrome. Collectively, these clinical studies with cirrhotic patients also suggest that enhanced circulating CO levels are associated with the development of the hyperdynamic circulatory syndrome.

2.1.3 Prostacyclin (PGI_2)

PGI_2 is generated by the activity of cyclooxygenase (COX) in endothelial cells and facilitates smooth muscle relaxation by stimulating adenylate cyclase to produce cyclic adenosine monophosphate (Claesson, et al. 1977) (Figure 4). There are two isoforms of COX. COX-1 is a constitutively expressed form, and COX-2 is an inducible form (Smith, et al. 2000; Smith, et al. 1996).

PGI_2 is an important mediator in the development of experimental and clinical portal hypertension (Hou, et al. 1998; Ohta, et al. 1995; Skill, et al. 2008). Increased COX-1 expression contributed to increased arterial vasodilation in the splanchnic circulation in portal hypertensive rats (Hou, et al. 1998). COX-2, however, was not detected in the superior mesenteric artery of those rats. These observations suggested that COX-1, not COX-2, would be responsible for the increased vasodilation in the superior mesenteric artery of portal hypertensive rats. However, inhibiting COX-1 only neither decreased PGI_2 levels nor ameliorated the hyperdynaic circulatory syndrome in portal hypertensive mice (Skill, et al. 2008). A study using both COX-1-/- and COX-2-/- mice in combination of selective COX-2 (NS398) and COX-1 (SC560) inhibitors, respectively, showed that blockade of both COX-1 and COX-2 ameliorated the hyperdynamic circulatory syndrome in portal hypertensive mice. Therefore, it is suggested that both COX-1 and COX-2 need to be suppressed to reduce PGI_2 production and to ameliorate the hyperdynamic circulatory syndrome (Skill, et al. 2008). Similar to experimental portal hypertension, circulating PGI_2 levels are also elevated in cirrhotic patients (Ohta, et al. 1995).

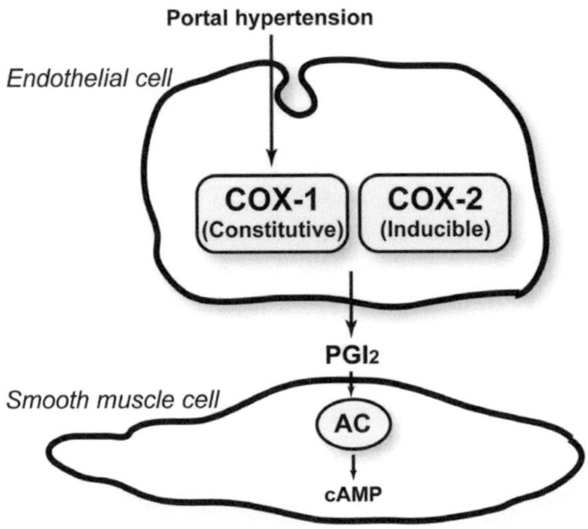

Fig. 4. Cyclooxygenase (COX) pathway in the arterial splanchnic and systemic circulation in cirrhosis and portal hypertension. COX-1 is a constitutive form, while COX-2 is inducible form. Both COX-1 and COX-2 seem to play a role in production of prostacyclin (PGI_2), which activates adenylate cyclase (AC) in smooth muscle cells to produce cyclic adenosine monophosphate (cAMP), thereby leading to vasodilation.

2.1.4 Endocannabinoids

Endocannabinoid is a collective term used for a group of endogenous lipid ligands, including anandamide (arachidonyl ethanolamide) (Wagner, et al. 1997). Endocannabinoids bind to their receptors, CB1 receptors, and cause hypotension (Figure 5). The bacterial endotoxin lipopolysaccharide (LPS) elicits production of endocannabinoids (Varga, et al. 1998) and thus develops hypotension.

Cirrhotic patients are generally endotoxemia, which is characterized by elevated endotoxin/LPS levels in the blood. Thus, it is not surprising that circulating anandamide levels are elevated in cirrhotic patients (Caraceni, et al. 2010; Fernandez-Rodriguez, et al. 2004). Cirrhotic rats also exhibit endotoxemia. Thus, antibiotic treatment to suppress endotoxemia decreased hepatic endocannabinoid levels and ameliorated the hyperdynamic circulatory syndrome in those rats (Lin, et al. 2011).

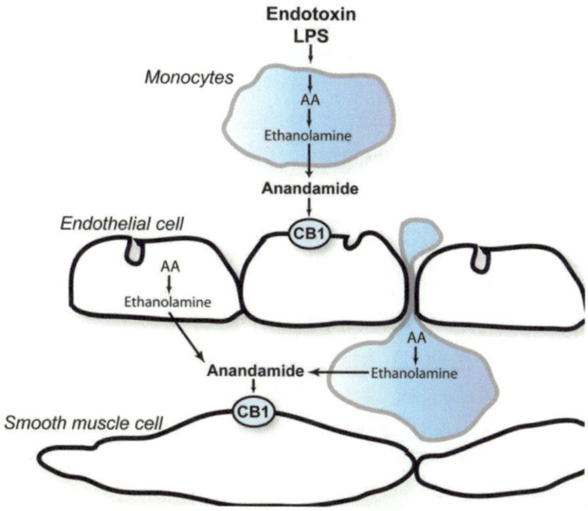

Fig. 5. Anandamide produced by circulating monocytes causes hypotension in cirrhotic rats and patients. Anandamide (arachidonyl ethanolamide) is an endogenous lipid ligand that belongs to endocannabinoids (Wagner, et al. 1997) and generated from arachidonic acid (AA). The bacterial endotoxin lipopolysaccharide (LPS) elicits production of anandamide in monocytes and endothelial cells (Varga, et al. 1998). Anandamide binds to CB1 receptors located on endothelial cells and smooth muscle cells and causes hypotension.

Monocytes and platelets are the two major sources of endocannabinoids in endotoxemia (Batkai, et al. 2001; Ros, et al. 2002; Varga, et al. 1998). When monocytes and platelets were pre-exposed to LPS and then injected to normal rat recipients, hypotension was developed (Varga, et al. 1998). Hypotension was however prevented by pretreatment of recipient rats with a CB1 receptor antagonist, SR141716A. Thus, endotoxemia elicits production of endocannabinoids in monocytes and platelets, leading to hypotension.

Anandamide levels were also elevated 2- to 3-fold and 16-fold in monocytes isolated from cirrhotic rats and patients, respectively, compared to their corresponding controls (Batkai, et al. 2001). Transplantation of monocytes isolated from cirrhotic rats or patients via intravenous injection, but not those monocytes from control rats, to normal recipient rats gradually caused the development of hypotension. In contrast, when normal recipient rats were pretreated with a CB1 receptor antagonist, SR141716A, the monocytes from the same cirrhotic rats or patients did not cause hypotension in those rats. Besides elevated anandamide levels, CB1 receptor levels were 3 times higher in hepatic arterial endothelial cells isolated from cirrhotic human livers than in those isolated from normal human livers. Importantly again, blocking CB1 receptor by SR141716A ameliorated arterial hypotension and the hyperdynamic circulatory syndrome in cirrhotic rats. Collectively, these results suggest that CB1 receptor can be a therapeutic target to ameliorate the hyperdynamic circulatory syndrome in cirrhosis and portal hypertension.

2.1.5 Endothelium-Derived Hyperpolarizing Factor (EDHF)

Endothelium-derived hyperpolarizing factor (EDHF) is also an important vasodilatory molecule that regulates vascular tone (Cohen 2005; Feletou & Vanhoutte 2006; Feletou & Vanhoutte 2007; Griffith 2004). It is associated with hyperpolarization of vascular smooth muscle cells and facilitates vasodilation. The term EDHF might be confusing, since it implies a single molecule (Feletou & Vanhoutte 2006). Currently, it is not still fully characterized what molecule EDHF is. However, accumulating evidence suggests that HDHF could be multiple molecules, including PGI_2 (Feletou & Vanhoutte 2006), NO (Cohen, et al. 1997; Plane, et al. 1998), epoxyeicosatrienoic acids (EETs) (Fleming 2004; Gauthier, et al. 2004; Li & Campbell 1997; Oltman, et al. 1998; Quilley & McGiff 2000; Widmann, et al. 1998), lipoxygenase [12-(s)-hydroxyeicosatetraenoic acid (12-S-HETE)] (Barlow, et al. 2000; Faraci, et al. 2001; Gauthier, et al. 2004; Pfister, et al. 1998; Zhang, et al. 2005; Zink, et al. 2001), hydrogen peroxide (H_2O_2) (Beny & von der Weid 1991; Chaytor, et al. 2003; Ellis, et al. 2003; Gluais, et al. 2005; Matoba, et al. 2002; Matoba, et al. 2003; Matoba, et al. 2000; Morikawa, et al. 2003; Shimokawa & Matoba 2004), potassium ions (K^+), C-type natriuretic paptides (Banks, et al. 1996; Wei, et al. 1994) and hydrogen sulfide (Mustafa, et al. 2011). It has also been suggested that EDHF function may be mediated through direct coupling between endothelial and smooth muscle cells at myoendothelial gap junctions composed of connexins (Cohen 2005; Feletou & Vanhoutte 2007; Griffith 2004) (Figure 6).

Most recently, a study by Mustafa et al. (Mustafa, et al. 2011) suggested that H_2S could be an EDHF. H_2S is synthesized endogenously from L-cystathionine-γ-lyase (CSE) and cystathionine-β-synthase (Hosoki, et al. 1997; Stipanuk & Beck 1982). The H_2S-mediated vasodilation occurs through the opening of ATP-sensitive potassium channel (K_{ATP} channel) and is independent of the activation of cGMP pathway (Zhao, et al. 2001). In the superior mesenteric artery of mice lacking CSE, hyperpolarization is virtually abolished. Most interestingly, H_2S covalently modifies (i.e., S-sulfhydrating) K_{ATP} channel and leads to relaxation of vessels.

EDHF seems to be more important in smaller arteries and arterioles than in larger arteries. This tendency has been recognized in a number of vascular beds, including mesenteric and cerebral arteries and arteries in ear and stomach (Tomioka, et al. 1999; Urakami-Harasawa, et al. 1997; You, et al. 1999).

It has not been established whether EDHF is involved in vasodilation and hypocontractility of arteries of the splanchnic and systemic circulation in cirrhosis and portal hypertension. Barriere et al. (Barriere & Lebrec 2000) reported that EDHF contributed to hypocontractility in the superior mesenteric artery isolated from cirrhotic rats when NO and PGI_2 production were inhibited. This hypocontractility was abolished when the vessels were further treated with inhibitors of small conductance Ca^{2+}-activated K^+ channel (SK channel), such as apamin and charybdotoxin, suggesting that EDHF blunts contractile response in cirrhotic rats (Barriere & Lebrec 2000). In contrast, a study by Dal-Ros et al. (Dal-Ros, et al. 2010) showed that the contribution of EDHF to vasodilation in mesenteric arteries was even smaller in cirrhotic rats than in normal rats. It was speculated that decreased expression of connexins (Cx), such as Cx37, Cx40, and Cx43, as well as Ca^{2+}-activated K^+ channel contributed to this smaller contribution of EDHF to vasodilation in the superior mesenteric

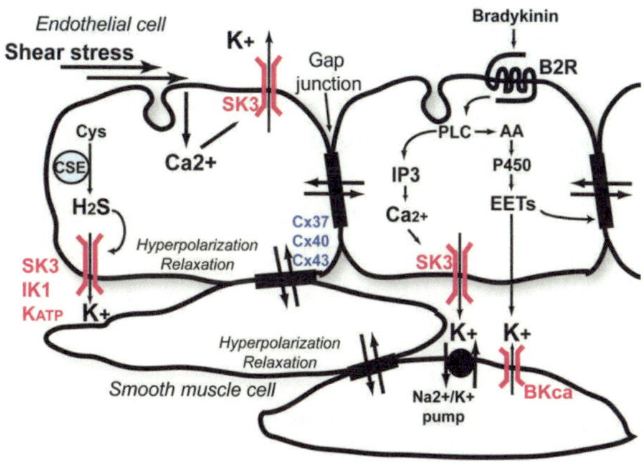

Fig. 6. Overview of endothelium-derived hyperpolarizing factor (EDHF) in the superior mesenteric artery. Shear stress generated by an increase in portal pressure increases endothelial Ca^{2+} concentration and produces hyperpolarization by activating ion channels, such as small conductance calcium-activated potassium channel (SK3) and intermediate conductance calcium-activated potassium channel (IK1). Hydrogen sulfide (H_2S) is formed in vascular endothelial cells from cysteine by L-cystathionine-gamma-lyase (CSE). H_2S causes hyperpolarization through activation of SK3, IK1 and ATP-sensitive potassium channel (KATP). Connexins (Cx) 37 and 40 are predominant gap junction proteins in endothelial cells and contribute to EDHF-mediated response. Connexin 43 (Cx43) is also present at the gap junction, but it does not play a major role in this context. Potassium ion (K+) activates Na+/K+-ATPase pump, preventing the effects of any substantial rise of potassium during endothelium-dependent hyperpolarization. Bradykinin, through its G-protein coupled receptor (B2R), activates the metabolism of arachidonic acid (AA) via cytochrome P450 monooxygenase (P450). Bradykinin also activates phospholipase C (PLC) that stimulates inositol trisphosphate (IP3) to increase cytosolic Ca^{2+} concentration. Epoxyeicosatrienoic acids (EETs) cause hyperpolarization/relaxation, acting through the voltage-gated potassium channel (BKCa) and gap junction.

artery of cirrhotic rats (Dal-Ros, et al. 2010). However, Bolognesi et al. (Bolognesi, et al. 2011) presented that mesenteric arteries isolated from cirrhotic rats exhibited elevated Cx40 and Cx43 expression, which increased sensitivity to epoxyeicosatrienoic acids (EETs) in those arteries and contributed to enhanced vasodilation.

2.1.6 Tumor necrosis factor α

A proinflammatory cytokine, tumor necrosis factor α (TNFα), is produced by mononuclear cells upon activation by bacterial endotoxins. In cirrhosis and portal hypertension, therefore, TNFα levels are elevated (Lopez-Talavera, et al. 1995; Mookerjee, et al. 2003). Inhibition of TNFα action by an anti-TNFα antibody resulted in a significant reduction in hepatic venous pressure gradient (HVPG) of patients with alcoholic hepatitis (Mookerjee, et al. 2003). Similarly, inhibition of TNFα synthesis by thalidomide also prevented the development of the hyperdynamic circulatory syndrome in portal hypertensive rats (Lopez-Talavera, et al. 1996). The mechanism of TNFα action in cirrhosis and portal hypertension is not fully understood.

TNFα stimulates NOS activity by increasing BH_4 production through stimulation of expression and activity of guanosine triphosphate-cyclohydrolase I, a key enzyme for the regulation of BH_4 biosynthesis in endothelial cells (Katusic, et al. 1998; Rosenkranz-Weiss, et al. 1994). Enhanced BH_4 production directly increases eNOS-derived NO production (Katusic, et al. 1998; Rosenkranz-Weiss, et al. 1994; Wever, et al. 1997). In biliary cirrhotic rats, it was demonstrated that TNFα, through the activation of iNOS in the aorta and lung, plays a role in the development of the hyperdynamic circulatory syndrome and the hepatopulmonary syndrome (Sztrymf, et al. 2004).

2.1.7 Adrenomedullin

Adrenomedullin is an endogenous vasodilatory peptide consisting of 52 amino acid residues in human and 50 amino acid residues in the rat (Kitamura, et al. 1993; Kitamura, et al. 1993; Nuki, et al. 1993). The major producers of circulating adrenomedullin are vascular smooth muscle cells (Sugo, et al. 1994) and endothelial cells (Sugo, et al. 1995). Adrenomedullin binds to and induces its signaling through the G-protein-coupled calcitonin receptor-like receptor/receptor activity-modifying protein (RAMP)2 and 3, which are expressed in multiple tissues, including blood vessels, kidney, lung, atrium, gastrointestinal tract, spleen, endocrine glands, brain and heart. Receptor RAMP2 is essential for angiogenesis and vascular integrity (Ichikawa-Shindo, et al. 2008). Adrenomedullin expression is up-regulated by hypoxia (Nagata, et al. 1999; Wang, et al. 1995) and inflammation (Sugo, et al. 1995; Ueda, et al. 1999), both of which are associated with neovascularization.

The vasodilatory action of adrenomedullin was considered in the beginning to be solely due to elevated cAMP production, i.e., endothelium-independent vasodilation. However, endothelial denudation substantially reduced its vasodilatory action in rodent aortic rings (Hirata, et al. 1995; Nishimatsu, et al. 2001). Furthermore, this adrenomedullin-induced endothelium-dependent vasodilation was exerted mostly through activation of the phosphatidylinositol 3-kinase (PI3-K)/Akt pathway (Nishimatsu, et al. 2001). It has been well established that this pathway is involved in various important actions in endothelial cells, such as activation of eNOS. While one study demonstrated in a mouse model of ischemia that adrenomedullin-induced collateral vessel formation in ischemic tissues was eNOS-dependent (Abe, et al. 2003), no study has so far shown that adrenomedullin activates eNOS through Akt activation.

Several studies have reported that in liver cirrhotic patients, circulating adrenomedullin levels are elevated and are associated with increased levels of plasma nitrite (a stable NO metabolite) and plasma volume expansion (Guevara, et al. 1998; Kojima, et al. 1998; Tahan, et al. 2003). Furthermore, the increased circulating adrenomedullin levels in those patients are inversely related to peripheral resistance (Guevara, et al. 1998). These observations indicate that adrenomedullin may promote excessive vasodilation and the hyperdynamic circulatory syndrome in cirrhotic patients. It is not surprising, therefore, that administration of an anti-adrenomedullin antibody prevented the occurrence of the hyperdynamic circulatory syndrome in the early sepsis (Wang, et al. 1998) and ameliorated blunted contractile response to phenylephrine in the aorta isolated from cirrhotic rats (Kojima, et al. 2004).

Portal hypertension alone, regardless of the presence of cirrhosis, increases adrenomedullin production. One clinical study showed that adrenomedullin and NO levels are elevated not only in patients with cirrhotic portal hypertension, but also in those patients with non-cirrhotic portal hypertension (Tahan, et al. 2003). How an increase in portal pressure influences production of adrenomedullin is an interesting and important question to be investigated.

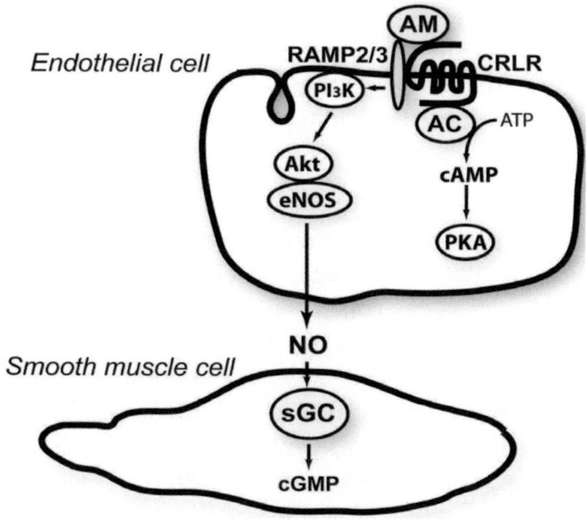

Fig. 7. Adrenomedullin causes vasodilation and hypotension. Adrenomedullin (AM) binds to and induces its signaling through the G-protein-coupled calcitonin receptor-like receptor (CRLR)/receptor activity-modifying protein (RAMP)2 and 3. The vascular action of adrenomedullin was at first considered to be solely due to elevated cAMP production by activation of adenylate cyclase (AC) in endothelial cells, thereby causing endothelium-independent vasodilation. Adrenomedullin-induced endothelium-dependent vasodialation is exerted mostly through activation of the phosphatidylinositol 3-kinase (PI3-K)/Akt pathway, which activates eNOS to produce NO. NO then diffuses into smooth muscle cells to activate soluble guanylate cyclase (sGC) and produce cyclic GMP (cGMP), leading to vasodilation.

2.1.8 Bradykinin

Bradykinin is a nine amino acid peptide and known to facilitate vasodilation (Antonio & Rocha 1962). Bradykinin leads to endothelium-dependent hyperpolarization through activation of phospholipase C (PLC), which could raise Ca^{2+} concentration and also stimulate production of EETs (Feletou & Vanhoutte 2006) (Figure 6). Bradykinin reduces sensitivity to glypressin (a long lasting vasopressin analogue) in both portal hypertensive and cirrhotic rats (Chen, et al. 2009; Chu, et al. 2000), thereby advancing vasodilation.

2.1.9 Urotensin II

Urotensin II is a cyclic peptide and has a structural similarity to somatostatin. It can function both as a vasoconstrictor and a vasodilator depending on vascular beds (Coulouarn, et al.

1998). In the systemic vessels including the aorta and coronary artery, urotensin II serves as the strongest vasoconstrictor known (Ames, et al. 1999; Douglas, et al. 2000). In rat mesenteric arteries, however, urotensin II causes vasodilation (Bottrill, et al. 2000). In biliary cirrhotic rats, plasma urotensin II levels were increased, and hypocontractility/vasodilatation was advanced in mesenteric arteries. An urotensin II receptor antagonist, palosuran, improved this hypocontractility/vasodilatation, by increasing RhoA/Rho-kinase expression and Rho-kinase activity (thereby more contraction) and decreasing nitrite/nitrate levels (Trebicka, et al. 2008). These observations may suggest that elevated levels of urotensin II also lead to hypocontractility/excessive vasodilation in the mesenteric arteries of patients with cirrhosis and portal hypertension. Thus, blocking the urotensin II-mediated signaling pathway may be an effective way to treat those patients.

2.1.10 Neuropeptide Y

Neuropeptide Y is a sympathetic neurotransmitter and known to cause α-adrenergic vasoconstriction (Tatemoto 1982; Tatemoto, et al. 1982). RhoA/Rho-kinase modulates various cellular functions such as cell contractility through phosphorylation of myosin light chain (Uehata, et al. 1997; Wang, et al. 2009). It was suggested that impaired RhoA/Rho-kinase signaling was responsible for excessive vasodilation and vascular hypocontractility in biliary cirrhotic rats (Hennenberg, et al. 2006). Acute administration of neuropeptide Y improved arterial contractility in the mesenteric arteries of cirrhotic rats by restoring impaired RhoA/Rho-kinase signaling (Moleda, et al. 2011). These observations may suggest that neuropeptide Y can be used for the treatment of hypocontractility/excessive vasodilation of the arterial splanchnic circulation in cirrhosis and portal hypertension.

2.2 Key factors

An increase in portal pressure alone can induce excessive arterial vasodilation and hypocontractility in the splanchnic and systemic circulation. In addition, chronic liver cirrhosis and portal hypertension are known to cause arterial wall thinning in these circulations. This arterial wall thinning is a critical factor that maintains excessive arterial vasodilation and hypocontractility and facilitates the development of the hyperdynamic circulatory syndrome in advanced portal hypertension.

2.2.1 Portal pressure

Using rats with partial portal vein ligation (Abraldes, et al. 2006; Fernandez, et al. 2005; Fernandez, et al. 2004; iwakiri 2011), which enables induction of different degrees of portal hypertension in animals (Iwakiri & Groszmann 2006), Abraldes et al. (Abraldes, et al. 2006) showed that portal pressure is detected at different vascular beds depending on the stage of portal hypertension. A small increase in portal pressure is first detected by the intestinal microcirculation. Then, further increased portal pressure is sensed by the arterial splanchnic circulation (e.g., the mesenteric arteries), finally followed by the arterial systemic circulation (e.g., the aorta). Thus, the intestinal microcirculation functions as a "sensing organ" to portal pressure. It is postulated that mechanical forces generated as a result of increased portal pressure, presumably cyclic strains and shear stress, activate eNOS and thus lead to NO production (Abraldes, et al. 2006; Iwakiri, et al. 2002; Tsai, et al. 2003).

When mild portal hypertension is generated in rats using partial portal vein ligation, an increase in portal pressure is too small to cause splanchnic arterial vasodilation. However, the level of vascular endothelial growth factor (VEGF) is significantly elevated in the intestinal microcirculation, followed by increased eNOS levels (Abraldes, et al. 2006). This model of mild portal hypertension may likely correspond to the portal pressure changes observed in early-stage cirrhosis, in which the progression of portal hypertension is generally slow. When portal pressure is further increased to a certain level, vasodilation develops in the arterial splanchnic circulation. Once vasodilation is established in the intestinal microcirculation and the arterial splanchnic circulation, arterial systemic circulatory abnormalities seem to follow (iwakiri 2011).

Like the above study using rats with partial portal vein ligation, portal pressure modulates intestinal VEGF and eNOS levels during the development of cirrhosis in rats (Huang, et al. 2011). We have shown that there is a significant positive correlation between portal pressure and intestinal VEGF levels ($r^2 = 0.4$, $p<0.005$). While plasma VEGF levels were significantly elevated in cirrhotic rats with portal hypertension (63.7 pg/ml, $p<0.01$) compared to controls (8.5 pg/ml), no correlation was observed between portal hypertension and plasma VEGF levels.

2.2.2 Arterial wall thinning

Endothelial NO plays a critical part in regulating the structure of the vessel wall (Rudic, et al. 1998). Studies using cirrhotic rats with ascites documented the occurrence of arterial wall thinning. Those rats exhibited decreased thickness of the vascular walls of the thoracic aorta, abdominal aorta, mesenteric arteries and renal artery (Fernandez-Varo, et al. 2007; Fernandez-Varo, et al. 2003). Administration of a NOS inhibitor significantly ameliorated wall thickness and attenuated the hyperdynamic circulatory syndrome, by increasing arterial pressure and peripheral resistance (Fernandez-Varo, et al. 2003). Since NO is predominantly derived from endothelial cells in these arteries, these observations suggest that increased eNOS-derived NO, at least in part, is responsible for this profound arterial wall thinning. Therefore, understanding the mechanisms of arterial wall thinning is important for the development of useful therapies for patients with portal hypertension.

3. Key molecules and factors – Portosystemic collateral vessel formation

In addition to excessive arterial vasodilation/hypocontractility in the splanchnic and systemic circulation, the formation of portosystemic collateral vessels is also thought to exacerbate portal hypertension (Bosch 2007; Iwakiri & Groszmann 2006). The portosystemic collateral vessel formation is probably an adaptive response to increased portal pressure, which, by releasing the pressure, may transiently help to delay the progression of portal hypertension. However, these collateral vessels eventually contribute to an increase in the blood flow through the portal vein and advance portal hypertension (Langer & Shah 2006). In addition, the formation of these vessels can also lead to detrimental complications. Since the vessels are fragile, they tend to rupture easily, causing esophageal and gastric variceal bleeding. Furthermore, since these vessels have the portal blood bypass the liver, toxic substances carried by it, such as drugs, bacterial toxins and toxic metabolites, returns to the systemic circulation and can cause portal-systemic encephalopathy and sepsis (Bosch 2007; Iwakiri & Groszmann 2006). The enlargement of pre-existing vessels as well as angiogenesis facilitate the development of these collateral vessels (Langer & Shah 2006; Sumanovski, et al. 1999). Studies have shown that vascular endothelial growth factor (VEGF) and placental growth factor (PIGF) play critical roles in the development of portosystemic collateral vessels in cirrhosis and portal hypertension.

3.1 Vascular Endothelial Growth Factor (VEGF)

The process of angiogenesis is regulated by growth factors exhibiting vasodilatory activity, such as VEGF. How are these angiogenic growth factors elevated in cirrhosis and portal hypertension? One mechanism may be initiated by an increase in portal pressure. As described previously, studies using portal hypertensive rats showed that a sudden increase in portal pressure is signaled to the intestinal microcirculation and induces intestinal VEGF expression (Abraldes, et al. 2006; Fernandez, et al. 2005). This sudden increase in portal pressure may create local mechanical forces, such as cyclic strains and shear stress, which may trigger VEGF induction.

It has been documented that administration of anti-angiogenic agents, such as blockers of VEGF receptor-2 (SU5416, anti-VEGFR2 monoclonal antibody) (Fernandez, et al. 2005; Fernandez, et al. 2004) and inhibitors of receptor tyrosine kinases (Sorafenib and Sunitinib) (Mejias, et al. 2009; Tugues, et al. 2007), reduces the formation of portosystemic collateral vessels and decreases portal pressure.

3.2 Placental growth factor

In addition to VEGF, placental growth factor (PlGF), another member of the VEGF family, has also been found to be increased in the intestinal microcirculation of portal hypertensive mice (Van Steenkiste, et al. 2009). In portal hypertensive mice lacking PlGF or given an anti-PlGF monoclonal antibody, both portal pressure and portosystemic collateral vessel formation were decreased. Collectively, these VEGF and PIGF studies suggest that blocking angiogenic activities, thereby decreasing the formation of portosystemic collateral vessels, has potential for the treatment of portal hypertension.

4. Summary

There are two major factors that contribute to excessive arterial vasodilation/hypocontractility in arteries of the splanchnic and systemic circulation in portal hypertension. One is an intrinsic factor and the other is a structural factor. The intrinsic factor includes vasodilatory molecules such as NO, CO, PGI_2, endocannabinoids, EDHF, adrenomedullin, TNFα, bradykinin and urotensin II. Decreased response to vasoconstrictors, such as neuropeptide Y, also facilitates hypocontractility of mesenteric arterial beds in cirrhosis and portal hypertension. The structural factor includes thinning of arterial wall (Fernandez-Varo, et al. 2007; Fernandez-Varo, et al. 2003). NO plays a critical role for arterial wall thinning in cirrhotic rats. However, its mechanism is not clear. In addition to excessive arterial vasodilatation/hypocontractility in the splanchnic and systemic circulation, the development of portosystemic collateral vessels is also regarded as the major factor that worsens portal hypertension (Bosch 2007; Iwakiri & Groszmann 2006).

4.1 Future direction

Both experimental and clinical studies of cirrhosis and portal hypertension have documented that a wide variety of molecules are involved in excessive arterial vasodilation/hypocontractility in the splanchnic and systemic circulation. This accumulation of knowledge allows us to further investigate molecular and cellular mechanisms in which these molecules exert excessive arterial vasodilation/ hypocontractility in cirrhosis and portal hypertension. In particular, it is interesting and important to address how changes in portal pressure, along with these molecules, influence the function and structure of vasculatures in the splanchnic and systemic circulation. Furthermore, it is not fully elucidated how these molecules are excessively induced in portal hypertension. Another important investigation would be to elucidate paracrine and autocrine regulations of vascular cells (e.g., endothelial cells, smooth muscle cells and fibroblasts) by these molecules. While the roles of these molecules in the vasculature per se have been described, few studies have investigated cell specific regulations and cell-cell communications exerted by these molecules.

Among those molecules introduced in this chapter, there are at least two molecules that are particularly anticipated for further investigation in the context of excessive arterial vasodilation and portosystemic collateral vessel formation in portal hypertension. One is hydrogen sulfide (H_2S). An increasing body of evidence suggests that H_2S is a crucial vasodilatory molecule in the superior mesenteric artery. However, it is not known whether H_2S is also involved in excessive arterial vasodilation in the splanchnic circulation in portal hypertension. Another molecule of interest is adrenomedullin. Studies using mice lacking adrenomedullin or its receptors indicated that adrenomedullin plays a critical role in the regulation of blood vessel integrity, including vascular stability and permeability (Caron & Smithies 2001; Fritz-Six, et al. 2008; Ichikawa-Shindo, et al. 2008; Shindo, et al. 2001). Given that increased vascular permeability and decreased vessel integrity are typical of vessels in cirrhosis and portal hypertension, this aspect of adrenomedullin should be explored in cirrhosis and portal hypertension.

5. Conclusion

To date, there are only limited options for the treatment of portal hypertension, despite the fact that portal hypertension leads to the most lethal complications of liver diseases such as gastro-oesophageal varices and ascites. Facing this situation, there is a strong need for studies of the vascular abnormalities associated with cirrhosis and portal hypertension (Shah 2009). These studies will have potential to lead us to develop novel targets for the treatment of portal hypertension.

6. References

Abe, M, M Sata, H Nishimatsu, D Nagata, E Suzuki, Y Terauchi, T Kadowaki, N Minamino, K Kangawa, H Matsuo, Y Hirata & R Nagai. (2003). Adrenomedullin augments collateral development in response to acute ischemia. *Biochem Biophys Res Commun*, Vol.306, No. 1, pp.10-5.

Abraldes, JG, Y Iwakiri, M Loureiro-Silva, O Haq, WC Sessa & RJ Groszmann. (2006). Mild increases in portal pressure upregulate vascular endothelial growth factor and endothelial nitric oxide synthase in the intestinal microcirculatory bed, leading to a hyperdynamic state. *Am J Physiol Gastrointest Liver Physiol*, Vol.290, No. 5, pp.G980-7.

Ames, RS, HM Sarau, JK Chambers, RN Willette, NV Aiyar, AM Romanic, CS Louden, JJ Foley, CF Sauermelch, RW Coatney, Z Ao, J Disa, SD Holmes, JM Stadel, JD Martin, WS Liu, GI Glover, S Wilson, DE McNulty, CE Ellis, NA Elshourbagy, U Shabon, JJ Trill, DW Hay, EH Ohlstein, DJ Bergsma & SA Douglas. (1999). Human urotensin-II is a potent vasoconstrictor and agonist for the orphan receptor GPR14. *Nature*, Vol.401, No. 6750, pp.282-6.

Angermayr, B, M Mejias, J Gracia-Sancho, JC Garcia-Pagan, J Bosch & M Fernandez. (2006). Heme oxygenase attenuates oxidative stress and inflammation, and increases VEGF expression in portal hypertensive rats. *J Hepatol*, Vol.44, No. 6, pp.1033-9.

Antonio, A & ESM Rocha. (1962). Coronary vasodilation produced by bradykinin on isolated mammalian heart. *Circ Res*, Vol.11, No. pp.910-5.

Arnold, WP, CK Mittal, S Katsuki & F Murad. (1977). Nitric oxide activates guanylate cyclase and increases guanosine 3':5'-cyclic monophosphate levels in various tissue preparations. *Proc Natl Acad Sci U S A*, Vol.74, No. 8, pp.3203-7.

Banks, M, CM Wei, CH Kim, JC Burnett, Jr. & VM Miller. (1996). Mechanism of relaxations to C-type natriuretic peptide in veins. *Am J Physiol*, Vol.271, No. 5 Pt 2, pp.H1907-11.

Barlow, RS, AM El-Mowafy & RE White. (2000). H(2)O(2) opens BK(Ca) channels via the PLA(2)-arachidonic acid signaling cascade in coronary artery smooth muscle. *Am J Physiol Heart Circ Physiol*, Vol.279, No. 2, pp.H475-83.

Barriere, E, Tazi, KA, Rona, JP, Pessione, F, Heller, J & D Lebrec, Moreau, R. (2000). Evidence for an endothelium-derived hyperpolarizing factor in the superior mesenteric artery from rats with cirrhosis. *Hepatology*, Vol.32, No. 5, pp.935-41.

Batkai, S, Z Jarai, JA Wagner, SK Goparaju, K Varga, J Liu, L Wang, F Mirshahi, AD Khanolkar, A Makriyannis, R Urbaschek, N Garcia, Jr., AJ Sanyal & G Kunos. (2001). Endocannabinoids acting at vascular CB1 receptors mediate the vasodilated state in advanced liver cirrhosis. *Nat Med*, Vol.7, No. 7, pp.827-32.

Beny, JL & PY von der Weid. (1991). Hydrogen peroxide: an endogenous smooth muscle cell hyperpolarizing factor. *Biochem Biophys Res Commun*, Vol.176, No. 1, pp.378-84.

Bolognesi, M, F Zampieri, M Di Pascoli, A Verardo, C Turato, F Calabrese, F Lunardi, P Pontisso, P Angeli, C Merkel, A Gatta & D Sacerdoti. (2011). Increased myoendothelial gap junctions mediate the enhanced response to epoxyeicosatrienoic acid and acetylcholine in mesenteric arterial vessels of cirrhotic rats. *Liver Int*, Vol.31, No. 6, pp.881-90.

Bosch, J. (2000). Complications of cirrhosis. 1. Portal hypertension. *Hepatology*, Vol.32, No. 1 Suppl, pp.141-56.

Bosch, J. (2007). Vascular deterioration in cirrhosis: the big picture. *J Clin Gastroenterol*, Vol.41 Suppl 3, No. pp.S247-53.

Bottrill, FE, SA Douglas, CR Hiley & R White. (2000). Human urotensin-II is an endothelium-dependent vasodilator in rat small arteries. *Br J Pharmacol*, Vol.130, No. 8, pp.1865-70.

Caraceni, P, A Viola, F Piscitelli, F Giannone, A Berzigotti, M Cescon, M Domenicali, S Petrosino, E Giampalma, A Riili, G Grazi, R Golfieri, M Zoli, M Bernardi & V Di Marzo. (2010). Circulating and hepatic endocannabinoids and endocannabinoid-related molecules in patients with cirrhosis. *Liver Int*, Vol.30, No. 6, pp.816-25.

Caron, KM & O Smithies. (2001). Extreme hydrops fetalis and cardiovascular abnormalities in mice lacking a functional Adrenomedullin gene. *Proc Natl Acad Sci U S A*, Vol.98, No. 2, pp.615-9.
Carter, EP, CL Hartsfield, M Miyazono, M Jakkula, KG Morris, Jr. & IF McMurtry. (2002). Regulation of heme oxygenase-1 by nitric oxide during hepatopulmonary syndrome. *Am J Physiol Lung Cell Mol Physiol*, Vol.283, No. 2, pp.L346-53.
Chaytor, AT, DH Edwards, LM Bakker & TM Griffith. (2003). Distinct hyperpolarizing and relaxant roles for gap junctions and endothelium-derived H2O2 in NO-independent relaxations of rabbit arteries. *Proc Natl Acad Sci U S A*, Vol.100, No. 25, pp.15212-7.
Chen, CT, CJ Chu, FY Lee, FY Chang, SS Wang, HC Lin, MC Hou, SL Wu, CC Chan, HC Huang & SD Lee. (2009). Splanchnic hyposensitivity to glypressin in a hemorrhage-transfused common bile duct-ligated rat model of portal hypertension: role of nitric oxide and bradykinin. *Hepatogastroenterology*, Vol.56, No. 94-95, pp.1261-7.
Chen, YC, P Gines, J Yang, SN Summer, S Falk, NS Russell & RW Schrier. (2004). Increased vascular heme oxygenase-1 expression contributes to arterial vasodilation in experimental cirrhosis in rats. *Hepatology*, Vol.39, No. 4, pp.1075-87.
Chu, CJ, SL Wu, FY Lee, SS Wang, FY Chang, HC Lin, CC Chan & SD Lee. (2000). Splanchnic hyposensitivity to glypressin in a haemorrhage/transfused rat model of portal hypertension: role of nitric oxide and bradykinin. *Clin Sci (Lond)*, Vol.99, No. 6, pp.475-82.
Claesson, HE, JA Lindgren & S Hammarstrom. (1977). Elevation of adenosine 3',5'-monophosphate levels in 3T3 fibroblasts by arachidonic acid: evidence for mediation by prostaglandin I2. *FEBS Lett*, Vol.81, No. 2, pp.415-8.
Cohen, RA. (2005). The endothelium-derived hyperpolarizing factor puzzle: a mechanism without a mediator? *Circulation*, Vol.111, No. 6, pp.724-7.
Cohen, RA, F Plane, S Najibi, I Huk, T Malinski & CJ Garland. (1997). Nitric oxide is the mediator of both endothelium-dependent relaxation and hyperpolarization of the rabbit carotid artery. *Proc Natl Acad Sci U S A*, Vol.94, No. 8, pp.4193-8.
Cosentino, F & ZS Katusic. (1995). Tetrahydrobiopterin and dysfunction of endothelial nitric oxide synthase in coronary arteries. *Circulation*, Vol.91, No. 1, pp.139-44.
Coulouarn, Y, I Lihrmann, S Jegou, Y Anouar, H Tostivint, JC Beauvillain, JM Conlon, HA Bern & H Vaudry. (1998). Cloning of the cDNA encoding the urotensin II precursor in frog and human reveals intense expression of the urotensin II gene in motoneurons of the spinal cord. *Proc Natl Acad Sci U S A*, Vol.95, No. 26, pp.15803-8.
Cruse, JM & RE Lewis, Jr. (1988). Cellular and cytokine immunotherapy of cancer. *Prog Exp Tumor Res*, Vol.32, No. pp.1-16.
Dal-Ros, S, M Oswald-Mammosser, T Pestrikova, C Schott, N Boehm, C Bronner, T Chataigneau, B Geny & VB Schini-Kerth. (2010). Losartan prevents portal hypertension-induced, redox-mediated endothelial dysfunction in the mesenteric artery in rats. *Gastroenterology*, Vol.138, No. 4, pp.1574-84.
De las Heras, D, J Fernandez, P Gines, A Cardenas, R Ortega, M Navasa, JA Barbera, B Calahorra, M Guevara, R Bataller, W Jimenez, V Arroyo & J Rodes. (2003). Increased carbon monoxide production in patients with cirrhosis with and without spontaneous bacterial peritonitis. *Hepatology*, Vol.38, No. 2, pp.452-9.

Dimmeler, S, I Fleming, B Fisslthaler, C Hermann, R Busse & AM Zeiher. (1999). Activation of nitric oxide synthase in endothelial cells by Akt-dependent phosphorylation. *Nature*, Vol.399, No. 6736, pp.601-5.

Douglas, SA, AC Sulpizio, V Piercy, HM Sarau, RS Ames, NV Aiyar, EH Ohlstein & RN Willette. (2000). Differential vasoconstrictor activity of human urotensin-II in vascular tissue isolated from the rat, mouse, dog, pig, marmoset and cynomolgus monkey. *Br J Pharmacol*, Vol.131, No. 7, pp.1262-74.

Ellis, A, M Pannirselvam, TJ Anderson & CR Triggle. (2003). Catalase has negligible inhibitory effects on endothelium-dependent relaxations in mouse isolated aorta and small mesenteric artery. *Br J Pharmacol*, Vol.140, No. 7, pp.1193-200.

Faraci, FM, CG Sobey, S Chrissobolis, DD Lund, DD Heistad & NL Weintraub. (2001). Arachidonate dilates basilar artery by lipoxygenase-dependent mechanism and activation of K(+) channels. *Am J Physiol Regul Integr Comp Physiol*, Vol.281, No. 1, pp.R246-53.

Feletou, M & PM Vanhoutte. (2006). Endothelium-derived hyperpolarizing factor: where are we now? *Arterioscler Thromb Vasc Biol*, Vol.26, No. 6, pp.1215-25.

Feletou, M & PM Vanhoutte. (2007). Endothelium-dependent hyperpolarizations: past beliefs and present facts. *Ann Med*, Vol.39, No. 7, pp.495-516.

Fernandez, M & HL Bonkovsky. (1999). Increased heme oxygenase-1 gene expression in liver cells and splanchnic organs from portal hypertensive rats. *Hepatology*, Vol.29, No. 6, pp.1672-9.

Fernandez, M, JC Garcia-Pagan, M Casadevall, C Bernadich, C Piera, BJ Whittle, JM Pique, J Bosch & J Rodes. (1995). Evidence against a role for inducible nitric oxide synthase in the hyperdynamic circulation of portal-hypertensive rats. *Gastroenterology*, Vol.108, No. 5, pp.1487-95.

Fernandez, M, M Mejias, B Angermayr, JC Garcia-Pagan, J Rodes & J Bosch. (2005). Inhibition of VEGF receptor-2 decreases the development of hyperdynamic splanchnic circulation and portal-systemic collateral vessels in portal hypertensive rats. *J Hepatol*, Vol.43, No. 1, pp.98-103.

Fernandez, M, F Vizzutti, JC Garcia-Pagan, J Rodes & J Bosch. (2004). Anti-VEGF receptor-2 monoclonal antibody prevents portal-systemic collateral vessel formation in portal hypertensive mice. *Gastroenterology*, Vol.126, No. 3, pp.886-94.

Fernandez-Rodriguez, CM, J Romero, TJ Petros, H Bradshaw, JM Gasalla, ML Gutierrez, JL Lledo, C Santander, TP Fernandez, E Tomas, G Cacho & JM Walker. (2004). Circulating endogenous cannabinoid anandamide and portal, systemic and renal hemodynamics in cirrhosis. *Liver Int*, Vol.24, No. 5, pp.477-83.

Fernandez-Varo, G, M Morales-Ruiz, J Ros, S Tugues, J Munoz-Luque, G Casals, V Arroyo, J Rodes & W Jimenez. (2007). Impaired extracellular matrix degradation in aortic vessels of cirrhotic rats. *J Hepatol*, Vol.46, No. 3, pp.440-6.

Fernandez-Varo, G, J Ros, M Morales-Ruiz, P Cejudo-Martin, V Arroyo, M Sole, F Rivera, J Rodes & W Jimenez. (2003). Nitric oxide synthase 3-dependent vascular remodeling and circulatory dysfunction in cirrhosis. *Am J Pathol*, Vol.162, No. 6, pp.1985-93.

Fleming, I. (2004). Cytochrome P450 epoxygenases as EDHF synthase(s). *Pharmacol Res*, Vol.49, No. 6, pp.525-33.

Fritz-Six, KL, WP Dunworth, M Li & KM Caron. (2008). Adrenomedullin signaling is necessary for murine lymphatic vascular development. *J Clin Invest*, Vol.118, No. 1, pp.40-50.

Fulton, D, JP Gratton, TJ McCabe, J Fontana, Y Fujio, K Walsh, TF Franke, A Papapetropoulos & WC Sessa. (1999). Regulation of endothelium-derived nitric oxide production by the protein kinase Akt. *Nature*, Vol.399, No. 6736, pp.597-601.

Furchgott, RF & JV Zawadzki. (1980). The obligatory role of endothelial cells in the relaxation of arterial smooth muscle by acetylcholine. *Nature*, Vol.288, No. 5789, pp.373-6.

Garcia-Cardena, G, R Fan, V Shah, R Sorrentino, G Cirino, A Papapetropoulos & WC Sessa. (1998). Dynamic activation of endothelial nitric oxide synthase by Hsp90. *Nature*, Vol.392, No. 6678, pp.821-4.

Gauthier, KM, JR Falck, LM Reddy & WB Campbell. (2004). 14,15-EET analogs: characterization of structural requirements for agonist and antagonist activity in bovine coronary arteries. *Pharmacol Res*, Vol.49, No. 6, pp.515-24.

Gauthier, KM, N Spitzbarth, EM Edwards & WB Campbell. (2004). Apamin-sensitive K+ currents mediate arachidonic acid-induced relaxations of rabbit aorta. *Hypertension*, Vol.43, No. 2, pp.413-9.

Gluais, P, G Edwards, AH Weston, PM Vanhoutte & M Feletou. (2005). Hydrogen peroxide and endothelium-dependent hyperpolarization in the guinea-pig carotid artery. *Eur J Pharmacol*, Vol.513, No. 3, pp.219-24.

Griffith, TM. (2004). Endothelium-dependent smooth muscle hyperpolarization: do gap junctions provide a unifying hypothesis? *Br J Pharmacol*, Vol.141, No. 6, pp.881-903.

Groszmann, RJ. (1993). Hyperdynamic state in chronic liver diseases. *J Hepatol*, Vol.17 Suppl 2, No. pp.S38-40.

Guevara, M, C Bru, P Gines, G Fernandez-Esparrach, P Sort, R Bataller, W Jimenez, V Arroyo & Rodes. (1998). Increased cerebrovascular resistance in cirrhotic patients with ascites. *Hepatology*, Vol.28, No. 1, pp.39-44.

Heinemann, A & RE Stauber. (1995). The role of inducible nitric oxide synthase in vascular hyporeactivity of endotoxin-treated and portal hypertensive rats. *Eur J Pharmacol*, Vol.278, No. 1, pp.87-90.

Hennenberg, M, E Biecker, J Trebicka, K Jochem, Q Zhou, M Schmidt, KH Jakobs, T Sauerbruch & J Heller. (2006). Defective RhoA/Rho-kinase signaling contributes to vascular hypocontractility and vasodilation in cirrhotic rats. *Gastroenterology*, Vol.130, No. 3, pp.838-54.

Hirata, Y, H Hayakawa, Y Suzuki, E Suzuki, H Ikenouchi, O Kohmoto, K Kimura, K Kitamura, T Eto, K Kangawa & et al. (1995). Mechanisms of adrenomedullin-induced vasodilation in the rat kidney. *Hypertension*, Vol.25, No. 4 Pt 2, pp.790-5.

Hosoki, R, N Matsuki & H Kimura. (1997). The possible role of hydrogen sulfide as an endogenous smooth muscle relaxant in synergy with nitric oxide. *Biochem Biophys Res Commun*, Vol.237, No. 3, pp.527-31.

Hou, MC, PA Cahill, S Zhang, YN Wang, RJ Hendrickson, EM Redmond & JV Sitzmann. (1998). Enhanced cyclooxygenase-1 expression within the superior mesenteric artery of portal hypertensive rats: role in the hyperdynamic circulation. *Hepatology*, Vol.27, No. 1, pp.20-7.

Huang, HC, O Haq, T Utsumi, S Sethasine, JG Abraldes, RJ Groszmann & Y Iwakiri. (2011). Intestinal and plasma VEGF levels in cirrhosis: The role of portal pressure. *J Cell Mol Med*, Vol.(in press), No.

Ichikawa-Shindo, Y, T Sakurai, A Kamiyoshi, H Kawate, N Iinuma, T Yoshizawa, T Koyama, J Fukuchi, S Iimuro, N Moriyama, H Kawakami, T Murata, K Kangawa, R Nagai & T Shindo. (2008). The GPCR modulator protein RAMP2 is essential for angiogenesis and vascular integrity. *J Clin Invest*, Vol.118, No. 1, pp.29-39.

Ignarro, LJ, GM Buga, KS Wood, RE Byrns & G Chaudhuri. (1987). Endothelium-derived relaxing factor produced and released from artery and vein is nitric oxide. *Proc Natl Acad Sci U S A*, Vol.84, No. 24, pp.9265-9.

Ishizuka, D, Y Shirai & K Hatakeyama. (1997). Duodenal obstruction caused by gallstone impaction into an intraluminal duodenal diverticulum. *Am J Gastroenterol*, Vol.92, No. 1, pp.182-3.

Iwakiri, Y. (2011). Endothelial dysfunction in the regulation of cirrhosis and portal hypertension. *Liver Int*, No.

Iwakiri, Y & RJ Groszmann. (2006). The hyperdynamic circulation of chronic liver diseases: from the patient to the molecule. *Hepatology*, Vol.43, No. 2 Suppl 1, pp.S121-31.

Iwakiri, Y, MH Tsai, TJ McCabe, JP Gratton, D Fulton, RJ Groszmann & WC Sessa. (2002). Phosphorylation of eNOS initiates excessive NO production in early phases of portal hypertension. *Am J Physiol Heart Circ Physiol*, Vol.282, No. 6, pp.H2084-90.

Jurzik, L, M Froh, RH Straub, J Scholmerich & R Wiest. (2005). Up-regulation of nNOS and associated increase in nitrergic vasodilation in superior mesenteric arteries in pre-hepatic portal hypertension. *J Hepatol*, Vol.43, No. 2, pp.258-65.

Katusic, ZS, A Stelter & S Milstien. (1998). Cytokines stimulate GTP cyclohydrolase I gene expression in cultured human umbilical vein endothelial cells. *Arterioscler Thromb Vasc Biol*, Vol.18, No. 1, pp.27-32.

Kitamura, K, K Kangawa, M Kawamoto, Y Ichiki, S Nakamura, H Matsuo & T Eto. (1993). Adrenomedullin: a novel hypotensive peptide isolated from human pheochromocytoma. *Biochem Biophys Res Commun*, Vol.192, No. 2, pp.553-60.

Kitamura, K, J Sakata, K Kangawa, M Kojima, H Matsuo & T Eto. (1993). Cloning and characterization of cDNA encoding a precursor for human adrenomedullin. *Biochem Biophys Res Commun*, Vol.194, No. 2, pp.720-5.

Kojima, H, S Sakurai, M Uemura, H Satoh, T Nakashima, N Minamino, K Kangawa, H Matsuo & H Fukui. (2004). Adrenomedullin contributes to vascular hyporeactivity in cirrhotic rats with ascites via a release of nitric oxide. *Scand J Gastroenterol*, Vol.39, No. 7, pp.686-93.

Kojima, H, T Tsujimoto, M Uemura, A Takaya, S Okamoto, S Ueda, K Nishio, S Miyamoto, A Kubo, N Minamino, K Kangawa, H Matsuo & H Fukui. (1998). Significance of increased plasma adrenomedullin concentration in patients with cirrhosis. *J Hepatol*, Vol.28, No. 5, pp.840-6.

Kwon, S, Iwakiri, Y., Cadelina, G., and Groszmann, RJ. (2004). Neuronal Nitric Oxide Synthase Plays a Role in the Vasodilation Observed in the Splanchnic Circulation in Chronic Portal Hypertensive Rats. *Hepatology*, Vol.40, No. 4, pp.184A.

Langer, DA & VH Shah. (2006). Nitric oxide and portal hypertension: interface of vasoreactivity and angiogenesis. *J Hepatol*, Vol.44, No. 1, pp.209-16.

Li, PL & WB Campbell. (1997). Epoxyeicosatrienoic acids activate K+ channels in coronary smooth muscle through a guanine nucleotide binding protein. *Circ Res*, Vol.80, No. 6, pp.877-84.

Lin, HC, YY Yang, TH Tsai, CM Huang, YT Huang, FY Lee, TT Liu & SD Lee. (2011). The relationship between endotoxemia and hepatic endocannabinoids in cirrhotic rats with portal hypertension. *J Hepatol*, Vol.54, No. 6, pp.1145-53.

Liu, H, D Song & SS Lee. (2001). Role of heme oxygenase-carbon monoxide pathway in pathogenesis of cirrhotic cardiomyopathy in the rat. *Am J Physiol Gastrointest Liver Physiol*, Vol.280, No. 1, pp.G68-74.

Lopez-Talavera, JC, G Cadelina, J Olchowski, W Merrill & RJ Groszmann. (1996). Thalidomide inhibits tumor necrosis factor alpha, decreases nitric oxide synthesis, and ameliorates the hyperdynamic circulatory syndrome in portal-hypertensive rats. *Hepatology*, Vol.23, No. 6, pp.1616-21.

Lopez-Talavera, JC, WW Merrill & RJ Groszmann. (1995). Tumor necrosis factor alpha: a major contributor to the hyperdynamic circulation in prehepatic portal-hypertensive rats. *Gastroenterology*, Vol.108, No. 3, pp.761-7.

Matoba, T, H Shimokawa, H Kubota, K Morikawa, T Fujiki, I Kunihiro, Y Mukai, Y Hirakawa & A Takeshita. (2002). Hydrogen peroxide is an endothelium-derived hyperpolarizing factor in human mesenteric arteries. *Biochem Biophys Res Commun*, Vol.290, No. 3, pp.909-13.

Matoba, T, H Shimokawa, K Morikawa, H Kubota, I Kunihiro, L Urakami-Harasawa, Y Mukai, Y Hirakawa, T Akaike & A Takeshita. (2003). Electron spin resonance detection of hydrogen peroxide as an endothelium-derived hyperpolarizing factor in porcine coronary microvessels. *Arterioscler Thromb Vasc Biol*, Vol.23, No. 7, pp.1224-30.

Matoba, T, H Shimokawa, M Nakashima, Y Hirakawa, Y Mukai, K Hirano, H Kanaide & A Takeshita. (2000). Hydrogen peroxide is an endothelium-derived hyperpolarizing factor in mice. *J Clin Invest*, Vol.106, No. 12, pp.1521-30.

Mayer, B & ER Werner. (1995). In search of a function for tetrahydrobiopterin in the biosynthesis of nitric oxide. *Naunyn Schmiedebergs Arch Pharmacol*, Vol.351, No. 5, pp.453-63.

Mejias, M, E Garcia-Pras, C Tiani, R Miquel, J Bosch & M Fernandez. (2009). Beneficial effects of sorafenib on splanchnic, intrahepatic, and portocollateral circulations in portal hypertensive and cirrhotic rats. *Hepatology*, Vol.49, No. 4, pp.1245-56.

Miyazono, M, C Garat, KG Morris, Jr. & EP Carter. (2002). Decreased renal heme oxygenase-1 expression contributes to decreased renal function during cirrhosis. *Am J Physiol Renal Physiol*, Vol.283, No. 5, pp.F1123-31.

Moleda, L, J Trebicka, P Dietrich, E Gabele, C Hellerbrand, RH Straub, T Sauerbruch, J Schoelmerich & R Wiest. (2011). Amelioration of portal hypertension and the hyperdynamic circulatory syndrome in cirrhotic rats by neuropeptide Y via pronounced splanchnic vasoaction. *Gut*, No.

Mookerjee, RP, S Sen, NA Davies, SJ Hodges, R Williams & R Jalan. (2003). Tumour necrosis factor alpha is an important mediator of portal and systemic haemodynamic derangements in alcoholic hepatitis. *Gut*, Vol.52, No. 8, pp.1182-7.

Morales-Ruiz, M, W Jimenez, D Perez-Sala, J Ros, A Leivas, S Lamas, F Rivera & V Arroyo. (1996). Increased nitric oxide synthase expression in arterial vessels of cirrhotic rats with ascites. *Hepatology*, Vol.24, No. 6, pp.1481-6.

Morikawa, K, H Shimokawa, T Matoba, H Kubota, T Akaike, MA Talukder, M Hatanaka, T Fujiki, H Maeda, S Takahashi & A Takeshita. (2003). Pivotal role of Cu,Zn-superoxide dismutase in endothelium-dependent hyperpolarization. *J Clin Invest*, Vol.112, No. 12, pp.1871-9.

Mustafa, AK, G Sikka, SK Gazi, J Steppan, SM Jung, AK Bhunia, VM Barodka, FK Gazi, RK Barrow, R Wang, LM Amzel, DE Berkowitz & SH Snyder. (2011). Hydrogen Sulfide as Endothelium-Derived Hyperpolarizing Factor Sulfhydrates Potassium Channels. *Circ Res*, No.

Nagata, D, Y Hirata, E Suzuki, M Kakoki, H Hayakawa, A Goto, T Ishimitsu, N Minamino, Y Ono, K Kangawa, H Matsuo & M Omata. (1999). Hypoxia-induced adrenomedullin production in the kidney. *Kidney Int*, Vol.55, No. 4, pp.1259-67.

Naik, JS & BR Walker. (2003). Heme oxygenase-mediated vasodilation involves vascular smooth muscle cell hyperpolarization. *Am J Physiol Heart Circ Physiol*, Vol.285, No. 1, pp.H220-8.

Nishimatsu, H, E Suzuki, D Nagata, N Moriyama, H Satonaka, K Walsh, M Sata, K Kangawa, H Matsuo, A Goto, T Kitamura & Y Hirata. (2001). Adrenomedullin induces endothelium-dependent vasorelaxation via the phosphatidylinositol 3-kinase/Akt-dependent pathway in rat aorta. *Circ Res*, Vol.89, No. 1, pp.63-70.

Nuki, C, H Kawasaki, K Kitamura, M Takenaga, K Kangawa, T Eto & A Wada. (1993). Vasodilator effect of adrenomedullin and calcitonin gene-related peptide receptors in rat mesenteric vascular beds. *Biochem Biophys Res Commun*, Vol.196, No. 1, pp.245-51.

Ohta, M, F Kishihara, M Hashizume, H Kawanaka, M Tomikawa, H Higashi, K Tanoue & K Sugimachi. (1995). Increased prostacyclin content in gastric mucosa of cirrhotic patients with portal hypertensive gastropathy. *Prostaglandins Leukot Essent Fatty Acids*, Vol.53, No. 1, pp.41-5.

Oltman, CL, NL Weintraub, M VanRollins & KC Dellsperger. (1998). Epoxyeicosatrienoic acids and dihydroxyeicosatrienoic acids are potent vasodilators in the canine coronary microcirculation. *Circ Res*, Vol.83, No. 9, pp.932-9.

Pfister, SL, N Spitzbarth, K Nithipatikom, WS Edgemond, JR Falck & WB Campbell. (1998). Identification of the 11,14,15- and 11,12, 15-trihydroxyeicosatrienoic acids as endothelium-derived relaxing factors of rabbit aorta. *J Biol Chem*, Vol.273, No. 47, pp.30879-87.

Plane, F, KE Wiley, JY Jeremy, RA Cohen & CJ Garland. (1998). Evidence that different mechanisms underlie smooth muscle relaxation to nitric oxide and nitric oxide donors in the rabbit isolated carotid artery. *Br J Pharmacol*, Vol.123, No. 7, pp.1351-8.

Quilley, J & JC McGiff. (2000). Is EDHF an epoxyeicosatrienoic acid? *Trends Pharmacol Sci*, Vol.21, No. 4, pp.121-4.

Ros, J, J Claria, J To-Figueras, A Planaguma, P Cejudo-Martin, G Fernandez-Varo, R Martin-Ruiz, V Arroyo, F Rivera, J Rodes & W Jimenez. (2002). Endogenous cannabinoids: a new system involved in the homeostasis of arterial pressure in experimental cirrhosis in the rat. *Gastroenterology*, Vol.122, No. 1, pp.85-93.

Rosenkranz-Weiss, P, WC Sessa, S Milstien, S Kaufman, CA Watson & JS Pober. (1994). Regulation of nitric oxide synthesis by proinflammatory cytokines in human umbilical vein endothelial cells. Elevations in tetrahydrobiopterin levels enhance endothelial nitric oxide synthase specific activity. *J Clin Invest*, Vol.93, No. 5, pp.2236-43.

Rudic, RD, EG Shesely, N Maeda, O Smithies, SS Segal & WC Sessa. (1998). Direct evidence for the importance of endothelium-derived nitric oxide in vascular remodeling. *J Clin Invest*, Vol.101, No. 4, pp.731-6.

Sacerdoti, D, NG Abraham, AO Oyekan, L Yang, A Gatta & JC McGiff. (2004). Role of the heme oxygenases in abnormalities of the mesenteric circulation in cirrhotic rats. *J Pharmacol Exp Ther*, Vol.308, No. 2, pp.636-43.

Sessa, WC. (2004). eNOS at a glance. *J Cell Sci*, Vol.117, No. Pt 12, pp.2427-9.

Shah, V. (2009). Therapy for portal hypertension: What is our pipeline? *Hepatology*, Vol.49, No. 1, pp.4-5.

Shah, V, R Wiest, G Garcia-Cardena, G Cadelina, RJ Groszmann & WC Sessa. (1999). Hsp90 regulation of endothelial nitric oxide synthase contributes to vascular control in portal hypertension. *American Journal of Physiology*, Vol.277, No. 2 Pt 1, pp.G463-8.

Shimokawa, H & T Matoba. (2004). Hydrogen peroxide as an endothelium-derived hyperpolarizing factor. *Pharmacol Res*, Vol.49, No. 6, pp.543-9.

Shindo, T, Y Kurihara, H Nishimatsu, N Moriyama, M Kakoki, Y Wang, Y Imai, A Ebihara, T Kuwaki, KH Ju, N Minamino, K Kangawa, T Ishikawa, M Fukuda, Y Akimoto, H Kawakami, T Imai, H Morita, Y Yazaki, R Nagai, Y Hirata & H Kurihara. (2001). Vascular abnormalities and elevated blood pressure in mice lacking adrenomedullin gene. *Circulation*, Vol.104, No. 16, pp.1964-71.

Skill, NJ, NG Theodorakis, YN Wang, JM Wu, EM Redmond & JV Sitzmann. (2008). Role of cyclooxygenase isoforms in prostacyclin biosynthesis and murine prehepatic portal hypertension. *Am J Physiol Gastrointest Liver Physiol*, Vol.295, No. 5, pp.G953-64.

Smith, WL, DL DeWitt & RM Garavito. (2000). Cyclooxygenases: structural, cellular, and molecular biology. *Annu Rev Biochem*, Vol.69, No. pp.145-82.

Smith, WL, RM Garavito & DL DeWitt. (1996). Prostaglandin endoperoxide H synthases (cyclooxygenases)-1 and -2. *J Biol Chem*, Vol.271, No. 52, pp.33157-60.

Sogni, P, AP Smith, A Gadano, D Lebrec & TW Higenbottam. (1997). Induction of nitric oxide synthase II does not account for excess vascular nitric oxide production in experimental cirrhosis. *J Hepatol*, Vol.26, No. 5, pp.1120-7.

Stipanuk, MH & PW Beck. (1982). Characterization of the enzymic capacity for cysteine desulphhydration in liver and kidney of the rat. *Biochem J*, Vol.206, No. 2, pp.267-77.

Sugo, S, N Minamino, H Shoji, K Kangawa, K Kitamura, T Eto & H Matsuo. (1994). Production and secretion of adrenomedullin from vascular smooth muscle cells: augmented production by tumor necrosis factor-alpha. *Biochem Biophys Res Commun*, Vol.203, No. 1, pp.719-26.

Sugo, S, N Minamino, H Shoji, K Kangawa, K Kitamura, T Eto & H Matsuo. (1995). Interleukin-1, tumor necrosis factor and lipopolysaccharide additively stimulate production of adrenomedullin in vascular smooth muscle cells. *Biochem Biophys Res Commun*, Vol.207, No. 1, pp.25-32.

Sumanovski, LT, E Battegay, M Stumm, M van der Kooij & CC Sieber. (1999). Increased angiogenesis in portal hypertensive rats: role of nitric oxide. *Hepatology*, Vol.29, No. 4, pp.1044-9.

Sztrymf, B, A Rabiller, H Nunes, L Savale, D Lebrec, A Le Pape, V de Montpreville, M Mazmanian, M Humbert & P Herve. (2004). Prevention of hepatopulmonary syndrome and hyperdynamic state by pentoxifylline in cirrhotic rats. *Eur Respir J*, Vol.23, No. 5, pp.752-8.

Tahan, V, E Avsar, C Karaca, E Uslu, F Eren, S Aydin, H Uzun, HO Hamzaoglu, F Besisik, C Kalayci, A Okten & N Tozun. (2003). Adrenomedullin in cirrhotic and non-cirrhotic portal hypertension. *World J Gastroenterol*, Vol.9, No. 10, pp.2325-7.

Tarquini, R, E Masini, G La Villa, G Barletta, M Novelli, R Mastroianni, RG Romanelli, F Vizzutti, U Santosuosso & G Laffi. (2009). Increased plasma carbon monoxide in patients with viral cirrhosis and hyperdynamic circulation. *Am J Gastroenterol*, Vol.104, No. 4, pp.891-7.

Tatemoto, K. (1982). Isolation and characterization of peptide YY (PYY), a candidate gut hormone that inhibits pancreatic exocrine secretion. *Proc Natl Acad Sci U S A*, Vol.79, No. 8, pp.2514-8.

Tatemoto, K, M Carlquist & V Mutt. (1982). Neuropeptide Y--a novel brain peptide with structural similarities to peptide YY and pancreatic polypeptide. *Nature*, Vol.296, No. 5858, pp.659-60.

Tomioka, H, Y Hattori, M Fukao, A Sato, M Liu, I Sakuma, A Kitabatake & M Kanno. (1999). Relaxation in different-sized rat blood vessels mediated by endothelium-derived hyperpolarizing factor: importance of processes mediating precontractions. *J Vasc Res*, Vol.36, No. 4, pp.311-20.

Trebicka, J, L Leifeld, M Hennenberg, E Biecker, A Eckhardt, N Fischer, AS Probsting, C Clemens, F Lammert, T Sauerbruch & J Heller. (2008). Hemodynamic effects of urotensin II and its specific receptor antagonist palosuran in cirrhotic rats. *Hepatology*, Vol.47, No. 4, pp.1264-76.

Tsai, MH, Y Iwakiri, G Cadelina, WC Sessa & RJ Groszmann. (2003). Mesenteric vasoconstriction triggers nitric oxide overproduction in the superior mesenteric artery of portal hypertensive rats. *Gastroenterology*, Vol.125, No. 5, pp.1452-61.

Tugues, S, G Fernandez-Varo, J Munoz-Luque, J Ros, V Arroyo, J Rodes, SL Friedman, P Carmeliet, W Jimenez & M Morales-Ruiz. (2007). Antiangiogenic treatment with sunitinib ameliorates inflammatory infiltrate, fibrosis, and portal pressure in cirrhotic rats. *Hepatology*, Vol.46, No. 6, pp.1919-26.

Ueda, S, K Nishio, N Minamino, A Kubo, Y Akai, K Kangawa, H Matsuo, Y Fujimura, A Yoshioka, K Masui, N Doi, Y Murao & S Miyamoto. (1999). Increased plasma levels of adrenomedullin in patients with systemic inflammatory response syndrome. *Am J Respir Crit Care Med*, Vol.160, No. 1, pp.132-6.

Uehata, M, T Ishizaki, H Satoh, T Ono, T Kawahara, T Morishita, H Tamakawa, K Yamagami, J Inui, M Maekawa & S Narumiya. (1997). Calcium sensitization of smooth muscle mediated by a Rho-associated protein kinase in hypertension. *Nature*, Vol.389, No. 6654, pp.990-4.

Urakami-Harasawa, L, H Shimokawa, M Nakashima, K Egashira & A Takeshita. (1997). Importance of endothelium-derived hyperpolarizing factor in human arteries. *J Clin Invest*, Vol.100, No. 11, pp.2793-9.

Van Steenkiste, C, A Geerts, E Vanheule, H Van Vlierberghe, F De Vos, K Olievier, C Casteleyn, D Laukens, M De Vos, JM Stassen, P Carmeliet & I Colle. (2009). Role of placental growth factor in mesenteric neoangiogenesis in a mouse model of portal hypertension. *Gastroenterology*, Vol.137, No. 6, pp.2112-24 e1-6.

Varga, K, JA Wagner, DT Bridgen & G Kunos. (1998). Platelet- and macrophage-derived endogenous cannabinoids are involved in endotoxin-induced hypotension. *Faseb J*, Vol.12, No. 11, pp.1035-44.

Wagner, JA, K Varga, EF Ellis, BA Rzigalinski, BR Martin & G Kunos. (1997). Activation of peripheral CB1 cannabinoid receptors in haemorrhagic shock. *Nature*, Vol.390, No. 6659, pp.518-21.

Wang, P, ZF Ba, WG Cioffi, KI Bland & IH Chaudry. (1998). The pivotal role of adrenomedullin in producing hyperdynamic circulation during the early stage of sepsis. *Arch Surg*, Vol.133, No. 12, pp.1298-304.

Wang, X, TL Yue, FC Barone, RF White, RK Clark, RN Willette, AC Sulpizio, NV Aiyar, RR Ruffolo, Jr. & GZ Feuerstein. (1995). Discovery of adrenomedullin in rat ischemic cortex and evidence for its role in exacerbating focal brain ischemic damage. *Proc Natl Acad Sci U S A*, Vol.92, No. 25, pp.11480-4.

Wang, Y, XR Zheng, N Riddick, M Bryden, W Baur, X Zhang & HK Surks. (2009). ROCK isoform regulation of myosin phosphatase and contractility in vascular smooth muscle cells. *Circ Res*, Vol.104, No. 4, pp.531-40.

Wei, CM, S Hu, VM Miller & JC Burnett, Jr. (1994). Vascular actions of C-type natriuretic peptide in isolated porcine coronary arteries and coronary vascular smooth muscle cells. *Biochem Biophys Res Commun*, Vol.205, No. 1, pp.765-71.

Weigert, AL, PY Martin, M Niederberger, EM Higa, IF McMurtry, P Gines & RW Schrier. (1995). Endothelium-dependent vascular hyporesponsiveness without detection of nitric oxide synthase induction in aortas of cirrhotic rats. *Hepatology*, Vol.22, No. 6, pp.1856-62.

Wever, RM, T van Dam, HJ van Rijn, F de Groot & TJ Rabelink. (1997). Tetrahydrobiopterin regulates superoxide and nitric oxide generation by recombinant endothelial nitric oxide synthase. *Biochem Biophys Res Commun*, Vol.237, No. 2, pp.340-4.

Widmann, MD, NL Weintraub, JL Fudge, LA Brooks & KC Dellsperger. (1998). Cytochrome P-450 pathway in acetylcholine-induced canine coronary microvascular vasodilation in vivo. *Am J Physiol*, Vol.274, No. 1 Pt 2, pp.H283-9.

Wiest, R, G Cadelina, S Milstien, RS McCuskey, G Garcia-Tsao & RJ Groszmann. (2003). Bacterial translocation up-regulates GTP-cyclohydrolase I in mesenteric vasculature of cirrhotic rats. *Hepatology*, Vol.38, No. 6, pp.1508-15.

Wiest, R, S Das, G Cadelina, G Garcia-Tsao, S Milstien & RJ Groszmann. (1999). Bacterial translocation in cirrhotic rats stimulates eNOS-derived NO production and impairs mesenteric vascular contractility. *Journal of Clinical Investigation*, Vol.104, No. 9, pp.1223-33.

Wiest, R & RJ Groszmann. (1999). Nitric oxide and portal hypertension: its role in the regulation of intrahepatic and splanchnic vascular resistance. *Seminars in Liver Disease*, Vol.19, No. 4, pp.411-26.

You, J, TD Johnson, SP Marrelli & RM Bryan, Jr. (1999). Functional heterogeneity of endothelial P2 purinoceptors in the cerebrovascular tree of the rat. *Am J Physiol*, Vol.277, No. 3 Pt 2, pp.H893-900.

Zakhary, R, SP Gaine, JL Dinerman, M Ruat, NA Flavahan & SH Snyder. (1996). Heme oxygenase 2: endothelial and neuronal localization and role in endothelium-dependent relaxation. *Proc Natl Acad Sci U S A*, Vol.93, No. 2, pp.795-8.

Zhang, DX, KM Gauthier, Y Chawengsub, BB Holmes & WB Campbell. (2005). Cyclooxygenase- and lipoxygenase-dependent relaxation to arachidonic acid in rabbit small mesenteric arteries. *Am J Physiol Heart Circ Physiol*, Vol.288, No. 1, pp.H302-9.

Zhao, W, J Zhang, Y Lu & R Wang. (2001). The vasorelaxant effect of H(2)S as a novel endogenous gaseous K(ATP) channel opener. *Embo J*, Vol.20, No. 21, pp.6008-16.

Zink, MH, CL Oltman, T Lu, PV Katakam, TL Kaduce, H Lee, KC Dellsperger, AA Spector, PR Myers & NL Weintraub. (2001). 12-lipoxygenase in porcine coronary microcirculation: implications for coronary vasoregulation. *Am J Physiol Heart Circ Physiol*, Vol.280, No. 2, pp.H693-704.

2

Cystic Fibrosis Liver Disease

Andrew Low and Nabil A. Jarad
Department of Respiratory Medicine,
Bristol Royal Infirmary,
UK

1. Introduction

Cystic fibrosis (CF) is the most common fatal autosomal recessive disorder in the white population with a frequency of 1 in 2500 live births. Inherited defects in the cystic fibrosis transmembrane conductance regulator (CFTR) gene result in abnormal regulation of salt and water movement across membranes. The overall feature of CF is that secretions are dehydrated due to water deprivation of luminal surfaces. This is true for the sino-pulmonary tract, biliary tree and for reproductive tubes (vas deferens and fallopian tubes).

Lung involvement is the main cause of morbidity and mortality, but this abnormal gene results in a multisystem disease affecting the liver, pancreas, sinuses, bones and reproductive system. Since its recognition in 1938 when life expectancy was 6 months (Davis, 2006), advances in medicine and a multidisciplinary team approach to patient care have increased the life expectancy of this condition such that children born today could expect to reach their 50s (Dodge et al., 2007; UK CF Trust 2009; USCF foundation 2009). The changing course of the disease has resulted in increasing relevance of other organ systems such as the liver.

2. Epidemiology of CF Liver Disease

The incidence of CF liver disease (CFLD) varies significantly among previous studies ranging from 5-30%. This is probably due to variations in definition.

On the whole, CFLD can be classified into 3 stages:

1. Biochemical - manifested by impaired liver enzymes
2. Structural - as increased bile content in the liver tissues or fatty infiltration visualised on liver ultrasound studies
3. Decompensated liver disease - which includes portal hypertension, hypoalbuminaemia, ascites and impaired coagulation.

The authors of this chapter propose to call 'clinically significant disease' as hepatic abnormalities that necessitate treatment by pharmacological and non-pharmacological methods.

In one study by Nash et al (2008), 30% of CF patients were found to be affected by clinically significant CFLD. Clinically significant disease in this study was defined as biochemical abnormalities manifesting with raised liver enzymes and ultrasonographic evidence of structural changes, but not necessarily liver cirrhosis.

Post mortem analysis suggested that focal abnormalities in the liver tissues are commoner than was previously thought occurring in 25-50% of CF patients (Gaskin et al., 1988; Nagel et al., 1989).

The prevalence of CFLD changes with age. Unlike most CF-related complications, CFLD appears to decrease with age. The reason for this is not clear. In one study by Scott-Jupp et al (1991) on 1100 CF patients in the South and West of England, the prevalence of CFLD - as judged by the presence of an enlarged liver or spleen (or both) - was 4.2%. The age-related prevalence rose to a peak in adolescence, and then fell in patients over 20 years old. The authors concluded that the decrease in prevalence was not due to drop-out of those who died of CFLD as the proportion of fall in incidence was much greater than the expected mortality rate from CFLD.

Other studies have also found increasing prevalence with age through childhood to mid-adolescence with no significant increase thereafter (Colombo, 2007).

The prognosis of patients with a well-established CFLD also varies. Herrmann et al (2011) reported that 7.9% of patients over the age of 40 have portal hypertension. But with a 7 year median follow up, only 28% went on to develop ascites or variceal bleeding, and liver failure was a late event. Median survival after a first variceal bleed is 8.4 years. This favours well when compared to the general cirrhotic population where 1 year survival is only 34%. Hence in the absence of other markers of decompensated liver disease, bleeding may not necessarily be a marker of poor prognosis (Colombo, 2007).

Older studies suggested a much more benign course, but it is now the 3rd most common cause of death after ventilatory failure and organ transplant complications. It is therefore an important cause for concern. The overall mortality rate is reported to be 2.5% (Moyer and Balistreri, 2009), and is associated with a higher risk of overall mortality when compared to CF patients without liver disease (Gallagher et al., 2011).

3. Pathophysiology of CFLD

CFTR is expressed in the epithelial cells of the biliary tract, but not in the hepatic cells. The main feature of CFLD is destruction in the biliary duct. The impaired viscosity of bile, albeit expected, was not consistently reported in studies.

Factors that enhance destruction of the biliary tree may lie in the epithelial toxicity of retained bile salt (Westaby, 2000). Other factors leading to the development of steatosis (fatty liver) are not related to defects in the CFTR gene and remains poorly understood. It has been attributed to malnutrition, essential fatty acid deficiency, carnitine or choline deficiency or insulin resistance (Moyer and Balistreri, 2009). Another presumed factor is the impairment of the architecture of the pancreas that shares a common exit with the common bile duct (Westaby, 2000).

Development of CFLD, including portal biliary cirrhosis and multilobular cirrhosis, is attributable to the abnormal CFTR gene. This results in abnormal transport of Cl^-, HCO_3^- and H_20 at the apical membrane of cholangiocytes such that the regulation of fluid and electrolyte content of bile is altered. As a result, bile is more viscous in CF patients than in non-CF individuals as with other mucous secretions.

Bile flow is reduced and the obstruction of intrahepatic bile ducts causes damage to hepatocytes and cholangiocytes through periductal inflammation, bile duct proliferation and fibrosis in portal tracts. This also results in activation of hepatic stellate cells, production of collagen, and stimulation of bile duct epithelium to produce TFG-β which is profibrinogenic (Moyer and Balistreri, 2009).

Why some patients with early manifestations of CFLD go on to develop liver cirrhosis and why some do not remains unclear. Understanding these factors in longitudinal studies will help design strategies for management of early liver disease with the aim of halting its progression and obviating its complications.

4. Genetics of CFLD

More than 1500 CFTR gene mutations have been described (O'Sullivan and Freedman, 2009), but there is no evidence of a phenotype relationship with specific mutations in the CFTR gene. In one study, (Duthie et al., 1992) they did not identify a difference in the frequency of Delta F $_{508}$, G551 or R553X mutations and the presence of CFLD.

However the same group found that several human lymphocyte antigens (HLA) subtypes were more prevalent in patients with CFLD compared to those without (Duthie et al., 1995).

Genetics was assumed to play a role not only in the emergence of CFLD but also in its prognosis. However despite several studies reviewed by Moyer and Balistreri (2009), it remains unclear why only a small proportion of CF patients might develop liver disease, or why there was such variability in severity.

Genetic modifiers may be one way to answer this question. Modifier genes have shown to play a role by increasing susceptibility to the development of CFLD by up-regulating inflammation, fibrosis or oxidative stress. Identifying these genetic modifiers may allow identification of CF patients at risk of developing CFLD and thus allow early use of prophylactic measures (Colombo, 2007). ACE, SERPINA, CSTP1, MBL2, TGF-β1 have all been identified as potential gene modifiers but only the SERPINA 1 Z allele has been found to be strongly associated with CFLD and portal hypertension (Bartlett et al., 2009).

5. Hepatic manifestations in cystic fibrosis

There is a broad spectrum of hepatic manifestations in cystic fibrosis as described in Table 1 (Colombo, 2007). Of those described the most clinically relevant in CF is focal biliary cirrhosis which may extend into multilobular biliary cirrhosis.

The incidence of impaired liver enzymes is high, affecting around 65% of patients with CF (Bhardwaj et al., 2009). Frequently these abnormalities may be transient and could relate to drug treatments or intercurrent infections (Moyer and Balistreri, 2009). The majority will not progress to clinically significant disease despite elevations of serum alanine aminotransferase, aspartate transferase or gamma-glutamyl transferase of up to 2.5x the upper limit of normal (Herrmann et al., 2010).

Type of lesion	Clinical manifestation	Frequency (%)
Specific alterations ascribed to the underlying CFTR defect	Focal biliary cirrhosis	20–30
	Multilobular biliary cirrhosis	10
	Portal hypertension	2–5
	Neonatal cholestasis	Rare
	Sclerosing cholangitis	Rare
	Micro-gallbladder	30
	Cholelithiasis	15
Lesions of iatrogenic origin	Liver steatosis	23–67
	Drug hepatotoxicity	Undefined
Lesions reflecting the effects of a disease process that occurs outside the liver	Hepatic congestion	Rare
	Common bile duct stenosis	Rare

Table 1. Major hepatic manifestations in cystic fibrosis (adapted from Colombo, 2007)

Steatosis is currently considered benign in cystic fibrosis with no evidence of progression to cirrhosis, portal hypertension or hepatic decompensation (Debray et al., 2011), while gallbladder abnormalities such as microgallbladder and cholelithiasis are frequently asymptomatic and detected on ultrasound requiring no intervention (Moyer and Balistreri, 2009). These hepatic manifestations can however contribute to post prandial abdominal discomfort, abdominal pain and fatigue in CF patients. Abdominal pain and fatigue are highly common in CF patients occurring in 77% (Jarad, 2009) and 87% (Sarfaraz et al., 2010) of patients respectively in the authors' unit.

Development of liver cirrhosis is less common, occurring in up to 30% of patients. This includes focal biliary cirrhosis with around 10% of CF patients developing multilobular biliary cirrhosis. Fewer still progress to liver failure and portal hypertension which can be associated with hypersplenism and gastro-oesophageal varices (Colombo, 2007).

Variceal bleeding in well established CFLD occurs in 30% of all cases. However it should be regarded as a rare complication in the adult CF population.

This cohort with cirrhosis and established portal hypertension are also at increased risk of developing hypoglycemia, malnutrition, hepatic osteodystrophy and worsening pulmonary status through hepato-splenomegaly and ascites-induced diaphragmatic splinting and intrapulmonary shunting (Colombo, 2007).

6. Investigations

No single reliable test is available to diagnose CFLD. Diagnosis thus relies on a combination of clinical assessment, liver biochemistry and other investigations. Table 2 gives proposed diagnostic criteria which incorporate these (Debray et al., 2011).

Hepatomegaly is often how CFLD is detected through routine examination, however, in isolation this is rarely associated with advanced liver disease. The slight enlargement of the liver size as well as the descending edge of the liver can be due to a combination of chronic lung sepsis and lung hyperinflation both of which are common in patients with CF lung disease.

Consider CFLD if at least 2 of the following are present:

- Hepatomegaly confirmed by ultrasonography (US)
  - > 2cm below the costal margin below the midclavicular line
  - and/or splenomegaly on US
- Abnormal liver function tests above the upper limit of normal
  - transaminases (AST and ALT) and GGT
  - on at least 3 consecutive occasions over 12 months
  - and other causes of liver disease excluded
- US evidence of liver involvement, portal hypertension or biliary abnormalities
- Positive liver histology (biopsy may be helpful where diagnostic uncertainty exist)

Table 2. Diagnostic Criteria for CFLD (Debray et al., 2011)

Each individual element of these criteria has their limitations when considered in isolation.

Abnormal biochemistry as previously discussed can occur frequently and often transiently. The chronic use of prophylactic oral antibiotics such as flucloxacillin in patients with chronic lung infection of Staphylococcus aureus may account for this. Also, the administration of beta-lactam antibiotics for acute pulmonary exacerbation is known to be associated with transient increases in liver enzymes. There is thus a low sensitivity for raised liver enzymes without abnormal radiology and abnormal histology. In addition some patients with multilobular biliary cirrhosis may have normal liver biochemistry (Colombo, 2007).

Ultrasonography is non-invasive and inexpensive. It can be useful in distinguishing between fibrosis, cirrhosis, ductal abnormalities and fatty infiltration (Colombo, 2007). The additional use of duplex scanning also allows detection of portal hypertension and portosystemic collaterals (Herrmann et al., 2010). Changes seen on US tests are more specific than clinical or biochemical abnormalities, with US abnormalities often preceding these changes. However, a normal scan does not exclude the development of future disease. The test is limited by both intra and interobserver variability in sonographic assessment with a positive predictive value of a normal US of only 33% and a sensitivity of 57% (Debray et al., 2011).

Williams et al (1995) devised and validated a scoring system for the severity of CFLD. The scoring system included the appearance of liver parenchyma, liver edge and periportal fibrosis. The score was found to distinguish transient liver disease from well established disease. The scoring system also identified sub-groups of patients who were regarded to have a pre-cirrhotic liver. A prospective prognostic evaluation of this scoring system has not yet been performed.

Magnetic resonance imaging (MRI) is emerging as an important investigation of the abdomen in CF patients (Figure 1). In a case-control study, we found that the pancreas was absent in CF patients with and without diabetes compared to age matched non-CF patients with Type I diabetes mellitus (Sequeiros et al., 2010). In another study we also reported that the spleen size, as measured on MRI, is reduced in patients with CF-related diabetes compared to those without and compared to age-matched patients with type I diabetes without CF (Jarad et al., 2010).

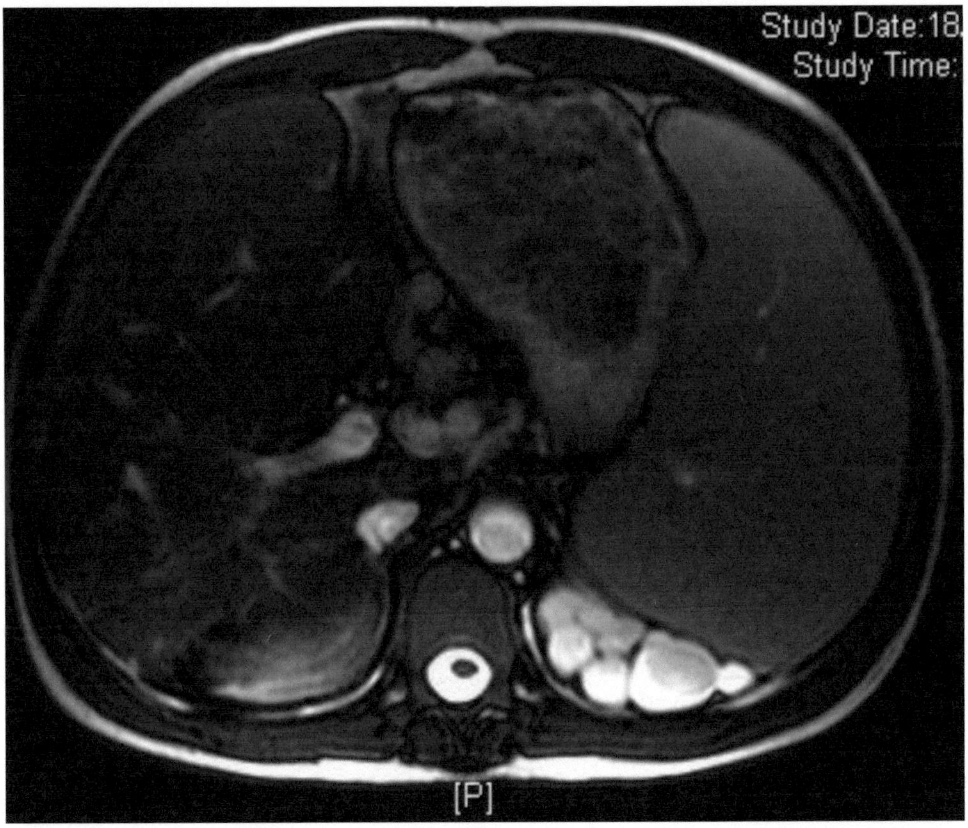

Fig. 1. MRI scan in a 24 year old lady with CFLD demonstrating liver cirrhosis, splenomegaly and tortuous veins on the spleen surface.

As for the liver, MRI scan is both a sensitive and a specific diagnostic test for CFLD. MRI can characterize the architecture of the liver structures (Westaby, 2000). A further delineation of the portal and splenic vascular bed and further enhancement of the definition of the liver architecture could be made through magnetic resonance cholangio-pancreatography (MRCP).

MRI and MRCP are non-invasive and well tolerated procedures, but the imaging remains too costly for the tests to become a screening procedure or to be used for follow-up purposes of all CF patients.

The presence of fibrosis on liver biopsy is both diagnostic and predictive of development of future portal hypertension and significant liver disease (Lewindon et al., 2011). However, the patchy distribution of lesions found in CFLD mean this invasive test can underestimate severity which limits its use (Colombo, 2007). It is thus not a routine test in many units unlike in chronic liver disease that is not linked to cystic fibrosis.

These limitations mean that CFLD often remains undetected until advanced stages prompting the need for other investigations. Both MRI and CT imaging can be useful in discriminating steatosis from fibrosis. MRCP and hepatic scintigraphy may help detect extra and intrahepatic biliary tree abnormalities in patients without clinically apparent disease and aid assessment of biliary drainage (Herrmann et al., 2010). These may play an important role in the future of CFLD. Other potential methods include transient elastography (fibroscan), which measures liver stiffness in a non invasive manner, which correlates closely with fibrosis and biochemical markers of fibrosis. Their value in CF remains to be determined (Debray et al., 2011).

A suggested approach to investigating CFLD and its initial management is shown in Figure 2.

Diagnosis of liver failure is similarly problematic due to the maintenance of liver function until the terminal phase. Clotting factors and prothrombin time should be monitored at least annually as this may give an indication. Liver failure should be considered if PT remains prolonged or if factors VII, X and II remain decreased despite vitamin K supplementation (Debray et al., 2011).

7. Management of CFLD

The mainstay of treatment for CFLD currently is optimisation of nutritional status and bile acid therapy - ursodeoxycholic acid (UDCA). The aim of the former is to avoid vitamin deficiency and malnutrition, though a proven benefit in CFLD is lacking (Herrmann et al., 2010).

UDCA is a bile acid that was shown to increase bile flow (Renner et al., 1980) and probably protects the hepatocellular structures from the harmful effects of hydrophobic bile ducts (Hoffman et al., 1990) by displacement of toxic hydrophobic bile acids, cytoprotection and stimulation of biliary bicarbonate secretion (Moyer and Balistreri, 2009).

Ultimately, the aim of UDCA is to delay progression of disease. There is evidence of improved liver biochemistry (Desmond et al., 2007) shortly after introducing UDCA and improved histological features of liver disease afterwards (Linblad et al., 1998). However, evidence of improved outcomes such as reduced need for transplantations or improved survival is lacking (Cheng et al., 2000). UCDA is widely used as it is the only available therapeutic agent and is generally well tolerated with few side effects. Recommended dosing is 20-30 mg/kg/day.

All patients with CFLD should receive annual liver assessment. The need for the yearly input of a gastroenterologist or hepatologist has been suggested (Debray et al., 2011). Though they may request intuitive tests and aid recognition of progression to cirrhosis, as well as complications such as portal hypertension, there is no evidence of superior outcome compared to a review by an experienced CF physician. This is important as CF patients are frequently seen in hospital and all receive an annual CF assessment. Adding an assessment by another discipline need only be introduced to a selected group of patients.

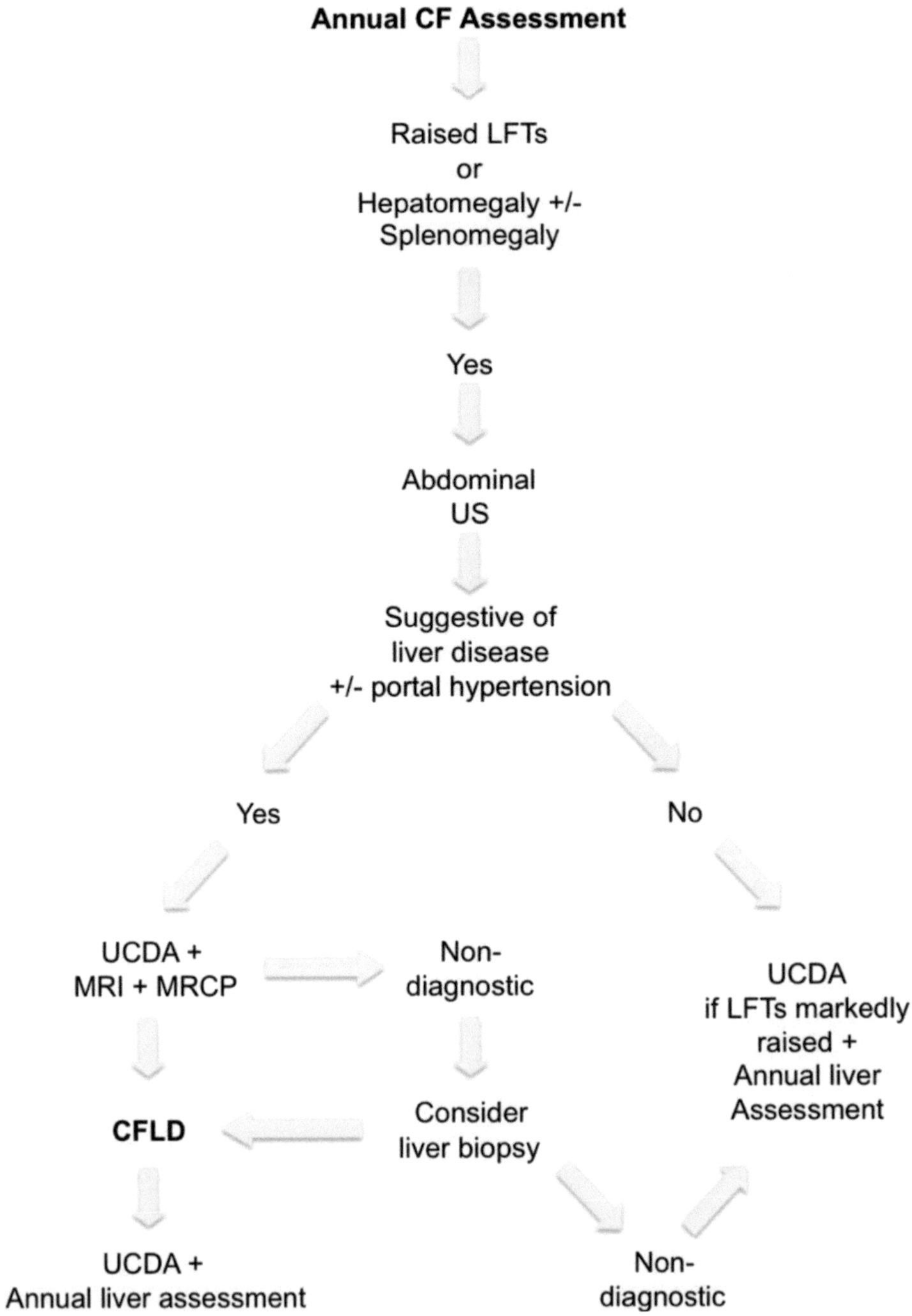

Fig. 2. Investigation and initial management of CFLD (adapted from Debray et al., 2011). Abbreviations: CF, cystic fibrosis; CFLD, cystic fibrosis liver disease; LFTs, liver function tests (i.e. liver enzymes including alanine transaminase, alkaline phosphatase; asparate transaminase and gamma glutamyl transpeptidase); MRCP, magnetic resonance cholangiopancreatography; MRI, magnetic resonance imaging; UCDA, ursodeoxycholic acid; US, ultrasound.

8. Management of portal hypertension

Though clear recommendations exist for non-CF patients with cirrhosis, there is no agreed guidance for this very different cohort of patients. Non-selective β-blockade is recommended, for example, which has not been evaluated in CF where lung disease may mean this is contraindicated. We do however use propranolol in at least 2 patients in our unit without significant respiratory side effects.

Band ligation is more effective than sclerotherapy, which can also carry a risk of bleeding both during and following the procedure which may result in repeated general anesthesia to the detriment of the patient's lung function. There is however no long term efficacy data in CF patients.

In the absence of such studies, recent guidance (Debray et al., 2011) states that all patients with cirrhosis and splenomegaly and/or signs of hypersplenism should receive an oesophagogastroduodenoscopy (OGD) every 2-3 years to screen for oesophageal varices. If large varices are detected these should be treated with band ligation and repeated until eradicated. Frequency of screening may need to be increased to annually. As with non-CF patients an OGD may be required more urgently in the presence of GI bleeding.

Transjugular intrahepatic portosystemic shunt (TIPSS) procedures have been used to achieve portal decompression to treat recurrent bleeding both pre-transplant (Colombo, 2007) and to allow long term survival (Herrmann et al., 2010). Surgical portal systemic shunting has also been used to preserve liver function, but carries this risk of acute liver failure and hepatic encephalopathy (Debray et al., 2011).

Rarely extra-pulmonary bleeding can occur from tortuous splenic and gastric veins (Figure 3). The efficacy of splenectomy and partial splenectomy remains unclear, with some studies suggesting this could stabilize lung function and delay progression of portal hypertension (Herrmann et al., 2010). Other studies exist reporting accelerated decline in lung function and no reduction in variceal bleeding (Debray et al., 2011) and hence it is not recommended currently. Thrombocytopenia and leucopenia due to hypersplenism requires no specific therapy.

9. Liver transplantation

Liver transplantation in end-stage liver disease is a viable option with encouraging results. There is evidence of improved lung function, nutritional status and quality of life (Columbo, 2007). Analysis of data from the United Network for Organ Sharing (UNOS) database by Mendezibal et al (2011) also demonstrated a survival benefit of liver transplant in CF when comparing those that had received a transplant to those that were still on the waiting list. The difference in mortality was significant in both paediatric and adult populations. Further analysis from UNOS shows good survival at 1 year and 5 years post transplant of 84% and 76% respectively (Arnon et al., 2011). This represents the largest review of outcomes following transplants for CFLD and supports the findings of previous smaller studies (Friedell et al., 2003; Melzi et al., 2006; Nash et al., 2008). However, overall survival post liver transplant for CFLD is less than that seen in non-CF patients who receive liver transplants for other indications. The most common cause of long term mortality is progression of pulmonary disease (Friedell et al., 2003), though haemorrhage also represents an important cause of death (Arnon et al., 2011).

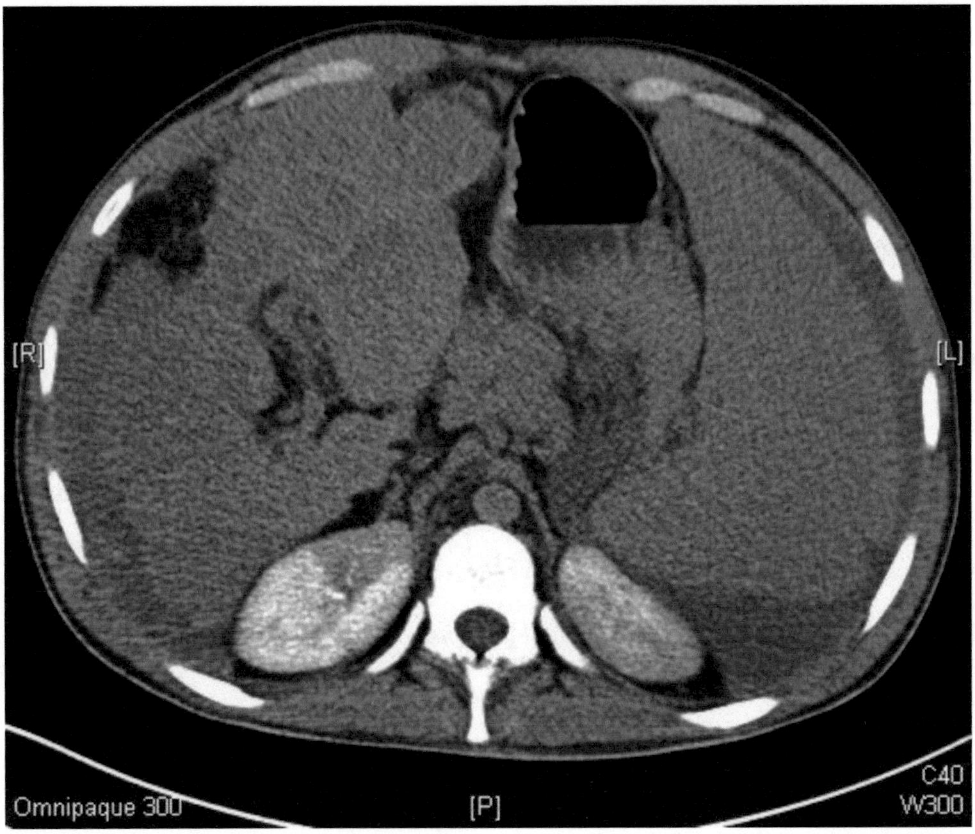

Fig. 3. CT scan in a 26 year old man with CF showing signs of liver cirrhosis, splenomegaly and haematoma around the spleen and within the abdominal cavity due to spontaneous splenic rupture. The patient died 1 week later.

The criteria and timing for liver transplantation remain uncertain. Although the criteria have widened with increased experience, inclusion of patients in liver transplantation needs to be evaluated on a patient-by-patient assessment. This is mainly because of concomitant lung disease, impaired nutrition (Figure 4) and of inability of some patients to withstand the rigor of transplant. One school of thought is that without signs of liver decompensation, survival is dependent on respiratory complications (Gooding et al., 2005). However, with other extra-hepatic benefits, earlier transplantation may be indicated. This needs to be weighed up against the risks associated with liver transplantation such as graft rejection and drug related complications (Debray et al., 2011).

Improved management options for the complications of portal hypertension may mean that transplantation ought to be considered in those with evidence of hepatocellular dysfunction in addition to portal hypertension, or those with rapidly deteriorating lung function. Other suggested indications include: the development of ascites and jaundice, intractable variceal bleeding, hepatopulmonary and portopulmonary syndromes, severe malnutrition unresponsive to intensive nutritio nal support, and deteriorating quality of life related to liver disease (Debray et al., 2011).

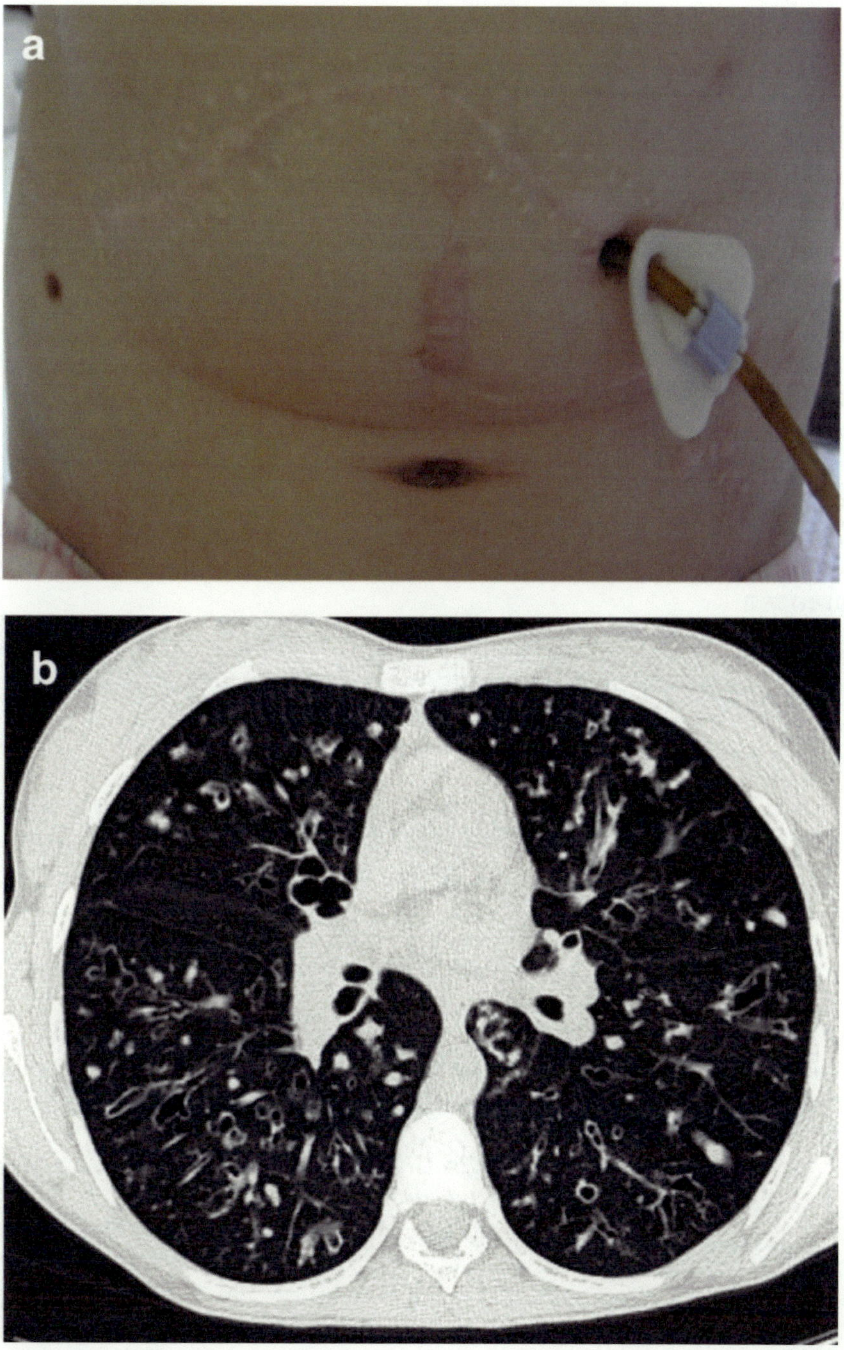

Fig. 4. a) A 21 year old female CF patient with liver transplant. Please note that the patient needed per entero-gastric (PEG) feeding due to concomitant malnutrition and low body mass index. b) Liver transplant was successful with little complication despite significant lung disease as seen by widespread bronchiectasis on her CT scan of the chest done several months after transplant.

In some occasions when patients may need both lung and liver transplant, it would be indicated to undertake transplantation of both organs. With the shortage of donated organs, this decision needs to be taken carefully. However, survival is comparable for combined liver and lung transplantation where this is indicated (Arnon et al., 2011).

10. Conclusion

CFLD occurs relatively frequently and is the most common non-pulmonary cause of mortality.

Improvements in the survival of cystic fibrosis patients mean that liver disease is likely to play an increasing role in long term morbidity and mortality. Current diagnosis relies on a combination of clinical examination and biochemistry, with old and new imaging techniques. UDCA is currently the only therapeutic option in CFLD, though its benefits on long term outcomes are not proven. Options addressing the complications of portal hypertension include TIPSS and OGD with variceal ligation. Orthostatic liver transplantation is also an option in end-stage liver disease with encouraging results.

11. References

Arnon, R., Annunziato, R. A., Miloh, T., Padilla, M., Sogawa, H., Batemarco, L., Willis, A., Suchy, F. and Kerkar, N. (2011) Liver and combined lung and liver transplantation for cystic fibrosis: Analysis of the UNOS database, *Pediatric Transplantation,* 15(3), 254-264.

Bartlett, J. R., Friedman, K. J., Ling, S. C., Pace, R. G., Bell, S. C., Bourke, B., Castaldo, G., Castellani, C., Cipolli, M., Colombo, C., Colombo, J. L., Debray, D., Fernandez, A., Lacaille, F., Macek, M., Rowland, M., Salvatore, F., Taylor, C. J., Wainwright, C., Wilschanski, M., Zemkova, D., Hannah, W. B., Phillips, M. J., Corey, M., Zielenski, J., Dorfman, R., Wang, Y. F., Zou, F., Silverman, L. M., Drumm, M. L., Wright, F. A., Lange, E. M., Durie, P. R., Knowles, M. R. and Gene Modifier Study, G. (2009) Genetic Modifiers of Liver Disease in Cystic Fibrosis, *Journal of the American Medical Association,* 302(10), 1076-1083.

Bhardwaj, S., Canlas, K., Kahi, C., Temkit, M., Molleston, J., Ober, M., Howenstine, M. and Kwo, P. Y. (2009) Hepatobiliary Abnormalities and Disease in Cystic Fibrosis Epidemiology and Outcomes Through Adulthood, *Journal of Clinical Gastroenterology,* 43(9), 858-864.

Cheng, K., Ashby, D. and Smyth, R. (2000) Ursodeoxycholic acid for cystic fibrosis-related liver disease. *Cochrane Database Syst Rev,*(2), p.CD000222.

Colombo, C. (2007) Liver disease in cystic fibrosis. *Current Opinion in Pulmonary Medicine,* 13(6) Nov, pp.529-536.

Davis, P. B. (2006). Cystic fibrosis since 1938. *Am J Respir Crit Care Med,* 173(5) Mar, pp.475-82.

Debray, D., Kelly, D., Houwen, R., Strandvik, B. and Colombo, C. (2011) Best practice guidance for the diagnosis and management of cystic fibrosis-associated liver disease, *J Cyst Fibros,* 10 Suppl 2, S29-36.

Desmond, C. P., Wilson, J., Bailey, M., Clark, D. and Roberts, S. K. (2007) The benign course of liver disease in adults with cystic fibrosis and the effect of ursodeoxycholic acid, *Liver International,* 27(10), 1402-1408.

Dodge, J. A., et al. (2007). Cystic fibrosis mortality and survival in the UK: 1947-2003. *Eur Respir J*, 29(3) Mar, pp.522-6.

Duthie, A., Doherty, D. G., Williams, C., Scott-Jupp, R., Warner, J. O., Tanner, M. S., Williamson, R. and Mowat, A. P. (1992) Genotype analysis for delta F508, G551D and R553X mutations in children and young adults with cystic fibrosis with and without chronic liver disease, *Hepatology*, 15(4), 660-4.

Duthie, A., Doherty, D. G., Donaldson, P. T., Scott-Jupp, R., Tanner, M. S., Eddleston, A. L. and Mowat, A. P. (1995) The major histocompatibility complex influences the development of chronic liver disease in male children and young adults with cystic fibrosis, *J Hepatol*, 23(5), 532-7.

Fridell, J. A., Bond, G. J., Mazariegos, G. V., Orenstein, D. M., Jain, A., Sindhi, R., Finder, J. D., Molmenti, E. and Reyes, J. (2003) Liver transplantation in children with cystic fibrosis: a long-term longitudinal review of a single center's experience, *J Pediatr Surg*, 38(8), 1152-6.

Gallagher, C. L., Gallagher, C. G., O'Laoide, R., Canny, G., Hayes, R., Slattery, D., Greally, P., Daly, L., Durie, P., Broderick, A., McElvaney, N. G., Bourke, B. and Rowland, M. (2011) Cystic fibrosis liver disease: a ten year follow-up study, *Irish Journal of Medical Science*, 180, S4-S5.

Gaskin, K. J., Waters, D. L., Howman-Giles, R., de Silva, M., Earl, J. W., Martin, H. C., Kan, A. E., Brown, J. M. and Dorney, S. F. (1988) Liver disease and common-bile-duct stenosis in cystic fibrosis, *N Engl J Med*, 318(6), 340-6.

Herrmann, U., Dockter, G. and Lammert, F. (2010) Cystic fibrosis-associated liver disease. Best Practice & Research in Clinical *Gastroenterology*, 24(5) Oct, pp.585-592.

Hoffman, A.F. (1990) Bile acid hepatotoxicity and the rationale of UCDA therapy in chronic cholestatic liver disease: some hypothesis. In: *Strategies for the treatment of hepatobiliary disease*. Paumgartner, G., Barbara, L., Roda, E., Stiehl, A. (Eds.), pp. 13-33. Springer, ISBN 978-0-7923-8903-3, The Netherlands.

Jarad, N. A. (2009) Extra-pulmonary Manifestations of Cystic Fibrosis. In: *Oxford Desk Reference:Respiratory Medicine*, Maskell, N. and Millar, A. (Eds), pp 252-257, Oxford, ISBN 978-0199239122, England.

Jarad, N. A., Sequeiros, I. M., Hester, K., Callaway, M., Williams, A. J., Sund, Z., Powell, T. and Wong, F. S. (2010) The size of the spleen by magnetic resonance imaging in patients with cystic fibrosis; with and without diabetes--a novel observational study, *QJM*, 103(4), 237-42.

Lewindon, P. J., Shepherd, R. W., Walsh, M. J., Greer, R. M., Williamson, R., Pereira, T. N., Frawley, K., Bell, S. C., Smith, J. L. and Ramm, G. A. (2011) Importance of Hepatic Fibrosis in Cystic Fibrosis and the Predictive Value of Liver Biopsy, *Hepatology*, 53(1), 193-201.

Lindblad, A, Glaumann, H & Strandvik, B (1998) A two-year prospective study of the effect of ursodeoxycholic acid on urinary bile acid excretion and liver morphology in cystic fibrosis-associated liver disease, *Hepatology*, vol. 27, no. 1, pp. 166-74.

Mendizabal, M., Reddy, K. R., Cassuto, J., Olthoff, K. M., Faust, T. W., Makar, G. A., Rand, E. B., Shaked, A. and Abt, P. L. (2011) Liver transplantation in patients with cystic fibrosis: analysis of United Network for Organ Sharing data, *Liver Transpl*, 17(3), 243-50.

Moyer, K. and Balistreri, W. (2009) Hepatobiliary disease in patients with cystic fibrosis. *Current Opinion in Gastroenterology*, 25(3), pp.272-278.

Nagel, R. A., Westaby, D., Javaid, A., Kavani, J., Meire, H. B., Lombard, M. G., Wise, A., Williams, R. and Hodson, M. E. (1989) Liver disease and bile duct abnormalities in adults with cystic fibrosis, *Lancet*, 2(8677), 1422-5.

Nash, K. L., Allison, M. E., McKeon, D., Lomas, D. J., Haworth, C. S., Bilton, D. and Alexander, G. J. M. (2008) A single centre experience of liver disease in adults with cystic fibrosis 1995-2006, *Journal of Cystic Fibrosis*, 7(3), 252-257.

Nash, E. F., Volling, C., Gutierrez, C. A., Tullis, E., Coonar, A., McRae, K., Keshavjee, S., Singer, L. G., Durie, P. R. and Chaparro, C. (2011) Outcomes of patients with cystic fibrosis undergoing lung transplantation with and without cystic fibrosis-associated liver cirrhosis, *Clin Transplant*. doi: 10.1111/j.1399-0012.2010.01395.x

O'Sullivan, B. P. and Freedman, S. D. (2009) Cystic fibrosis, *Lancet*, 373(9678), 1891-904.

Renner, E. L., Lake, J. R., Cragoe, E. J., Van Dyke, R. W. and Scharschmidt, B. F. (1988) Ursodeoxycholic acid choleresis: relationship to biliary HCO-3 and effects of Na+-H+ exchange inhibitors, *Am J Physiol*, 254(2 Pt 1), G232-41.

Sarfaraz, S., Sund, Z. and Jarad, N. (2010) Real-time, once-daily monitoring of symptoms and FEV in cystic fibrosis patients - a feasibility study using a novel device, *Clin Respir J*, 4(2), 74-82.

Scott-Jupp, R., Lama, M. and Tanner, M. S. (1991) Prevalence of liver disease in cystic fibrosis, *Arch Dis Child*, 66(6), 698-701.

Sequeiros, I. M., Hester, K., Callaway, M., Williams, A., Garland, Z., Powell, T., Wong, F. S., Jarad, N. A. and Group, B. C. F. D. (2010) MRI appearance of the pancreas in patients with cystic fibrosis: a comparison of pancreas volume in diabetic and non-diabetic patients, *Br J Radiol*, 83(995), 921-6.

UK CF Trust (2011) UK CF Registry. Annual data report 2009. 31 Mar 2011 Available from http://www.cftrust.org.uk

USCF Foundation. Patient Registry Report 2009. Available from http://www.cff.org/UploadedFiles/research/ClinicalResearch/Patient-Registry-Report-2009.pdf

Westaby, D. (2000). Liver and biliary disease in cystic fibrosis. In: *Cystic Fibrosis 2nd Edition*, Hodson, M.E. and Geddes, D.M. pp 289-300, Arnold Publication:. ISBN-13: 978-0340742082, London

Williams, S. G., Evanson, J. E., Barrett, N., Hodson, M. E., Boultbee, J. E. and Westaby, D. (1995) An ultrasound scoring system for the diagnosis of liver disease in cystic fibrosis. *J Hepatol*, 22(5), 513-21.

3

Extra Hepatic Portal Venous Obstruction in Children

Narendra K. Arora and Manoja K. Das
The INCLEN Trust International, New Delhi, India

1. Introduction

Portal hypertension is the commonest cause of upper gastrointestinal bleeding in children and up to 30% of cases with upper gastrointestinal hemorrhage can be fatal. Extrahepatic portal venous obstruction (EHPVO) is the commonest cause of portal hypertension in children and also one of the common causes in adults in India and other tropical countries (Arora, 1998; Poddar, 2008; Poddar 2000). In India, EHPVO is responsible for portal hypertension in about one third cases of adults and more than half of the cases in children (Sarin 2002; Dilawari 1992). EHPVO is characteristically refers to obstruction in the trunk of portal vein and it can extend to its branches and even splanchnic veins. Unlike cirrhosis, in EHPVO, the liver function is normal. The causes of portal venous obstruction and risk factors for upper gastrointestinal hemorrhage in children with EHPVO are not clearly understood. Most of the bleeds are spontaneous and some may be preceded by febrile illness, ingestion of drugs. Management of EHPVO involves acute management of the bleeding, secondary prophylaxis and shunting to reduce the portal pressure. This chapter attempts to compile the available evidences on EHPVO in children with special reference to experiences from India.

2. Definitions and terminology

EHPVO indicates portal hypertension due to blockage in the portal vein before the blood reaches the liver. EHPVO is a distinct disease entity of primarily vascular in nature and not classically associated with association of a primary liver disease. Portal vein thrombosis, a known complication of liver cirrhosis, other systemic diseases and malignancy, is not generally included in the disease entity EHPVO. Over time, EHPVO terminology has replaced the use of portal vein thrombosis (PVT) as it does not exclude the intrahepatic portal vein thrombosis and does not include formation of portal cavernoma associated with portal hypertension.

Baveno V workshop consensus statement defined EHPVO as (De Franchis, 2010):

- EHPVO is defined by obstruction of the extra-hepatic portal vein with or without involvement of the intra-hepatic portal veins and does not include isolated thrombosis of splenic vein or superior mesenteric vein (SMV).
- EHPVO is characterized by features of recent thrombosis or of portal hypertension with portal cavernoma as a sequel of portal vein obstruction
- Presence of cirrhosis and/or malignancy should be stated.

3. Epidemiology

EHPVO is a common cause of portal hypertension in the developing countries (30-55% of all variceal bleeders) and is second to cirrhosis (up to 5-13%) (Arora, 1998; Valla, 2002). EHPVO is also the most common cause of upper gastrointestinal bleeding in children. It accounts for almost 70% of pediatric patients with portal hypertension (Yachha, 1996; Arora, 1998). Literature from different parts of India indicated that in children EHPVO is responsible for 54% of portal hypertension (Poddar, 2008). Most (85-92%) of the upper gastrointestinal bleeding in Indian children was result of portal hypertension due to EHPVO (Poddar, 2008; Yachha, 1996).

Investigators across India have consistently observed that EHPVO occurs commonly in children belonging to low and lower middle socio-economic strata attending public sector hospitals. Pediatric gastroenterologists practicing in private sector hospitals see such patients infrequently. During last 10-15 years, the number of EHPVO patients gradually appears to be dwindling even in public sector hospitals. Thus it appears that the disease may have something to do with the living condition of the families and with improving economic state of the families, disease may become less frequent.

4. Etiology and pathogenesis

4.1 Etiology

The etiology of EHPVO in children has not been well documented. There are many etiologies for EHPVO namely infections, surgical procedures, vascular interventions, abdominal trauma, dehydration, congenital anomalies have been postulated. EHPVO is considered to be heterogenous with regard to etiology and pathogenesis, and vary with respect to age and geographical location. The causes can broadly be of five types; infection and inflammation, portal vein injury, developmental anomaly, prothrombotic causes and idiopathic.

4.1.1 Infection

Omphalitis, neonatal umbilical sepsis, intraabdominal infection, post umbilical catheterization have been linked to development of EHPVO in children. Although it is documented that portal vein thrombosis may occurs in neonates having umbilical vein catheterization, but most of these thrombi resolve within a short period (Larroche, 1970; Thompson, 1964). It is also proposed that phlebosclerosis is primary as a result of infection and/or and inflammation followed by thrombosis as a secondary event (Stringer, 1994). But evidence on this linkage is not very strong in children with EHPVO.

4.1.2 Trauma and surgery

Umbilical vein cannulation, abdominal surgery, and abdominal trauma in childhood could also lead to EHPVO (Yadav, 1993).

4.1.3 Congenital anomaly

Congenital defects like web, valves in the portal vein, portal vein stenosis, atresia or agenesis have also been reported (Odievre, 1977). There may be presence of other cardiovascular system congenital defects.

4.1.4 Prothrombotic state

Hypercoagulable states like deficiencies of antithrombotic factors (protein-C, protein-S, anti-thrombin III) have been reported in children with EHPVO (Bhattacharya, 2004; Pinto, 2004; Koshy, 1984; Dubuisson, 1997). Absence of genetic mutations in EHPVO patients and normal levels of antithrombotic factors in their parents suggested that the deficiency of antithrombotic factors may not be primarily of genetic origin, but may be secondary to the low hepatic blood flow due to portal vein thrombosis (low synthesis) and portosystemic shunt (increased clearance or consumption) (Dubuisson, 1997; Sharma, 2006). Other conditions like polycythemia vera, dehydration have also been proposed as the causes of EHPVO.

4.1.5 Idiopathic

Despite all efforts, the etiology of blocked portal vein remains obscure in a large proportion of patients. In India the majority of cases (up to 90%) are categorized as idiopathic (Poddar, 2003). Probably this is due to want of detailed etiological work-up.

4.2 Pathogenesis

4.2.1 Portal vein changes

In EHPVO, usually the entire length of the portal vein is occluded with extension into the splenic vein and sometimes into the superior mesenteric vein. In small proportions only the terminus of the portal vein at the hilum is occluded. Mostly the site of blockage is at the portal vein formation and in small proportions the total splenoportal axis is blocked. In a report by our group among Indian children with EHPVO (n=88), blockage were observed at portal vein formation, entire portal vein, spleninc vein and entire splenoportal axis in 39%, 34%, 16% and 11% respectively (Arora, 2002). On gross examination, the original portal vein is difficult to identify as it is usually replaced by a cluster of variable-sized vessels arranged haphazardly within a connective tissue support, called as the portal cavernoma. In cases of shorter duration, cavernoma may not be there. The porto-systemic collaterals develop over time leading to development of verices at different places in the gastrointestinal tract, and at other places depending on the portal venous pressure and duration.

In EHPVO the blockage being presinusoidal, intrahepatic venous pressure is normal and intrasplenic pressure is increased. The hepatic blood flow is relatively normal as the portoportal collateral vessels enable bypassing the blocked area. The hepatic blood flow may be reduced if the collaterals are not enough. EHPVO is a hyperkinetic circulatory state with increased cardiac output as a result of extensive porto-systemic venous collaterals.

4.2.2 Liver changes

Classically, in EHPVO cases liver is normal and the architectural pattern is preserved. Histopathology may reveal concentric condensation of reticulin fibers around portal tracts, sometimes extending into the parenchyma. Altered hepatic storage capacity and transport maximum for bromsulphalin and liodocaine (MEGX) excretion has been reported in EHPVO. Usually liver biopsy is not required in EHPVO cases, unless liver functions are deranged.

5. Clinical presentations

In children, EHPVO may manifest at any age beyond the neonatal period. EHPVO can present in two clinical forms: recent or acute and chronic. The clinical presentation also differs in children and adults.

5.1 Recent or acute EHPVO

This can present with abdominal pain, ascites or fever. This may, however, be asymptomatic and go unnoticed. In recent EHPVO, there is no evidence of porto-systemic collaterals and portal cavernoma. The extent of obstruction in portal vein and speed of evolution of thrombosis predicts the clinical manifestation. If associated with infection, features of sepsis may be there. But many a times these may be passed as episodes of acute abdomen or sepsis.

5.2 Chronic EHPVO

Most of the EHPVO present as chronic cases with the typical presenting symptoms like episodes of variceal or gastrointestinal bleeding, lump in the abdomen and hypersplenism.

EHPVO in childhood is most often chronic and presents with features of variceal bleeding and splenomegaly, whereas in adults it could be either acute or chronic.

5.2.1 Variceal bleeding

Esophageal varices are the most common site of variceal bleeding. The majority of children (85% to 90%) with EHPVO present with variceal bleeding (Arora, 1998; Poddar, 2008; Valla, 2002). The usual presentation for children with EHPVO is sudden, unexpected and, often, massive hemetemesis. Bleeding usually occurs in first or second decade of life. Some of the children also present with recurrent, well-tolerated bleeds with variable degree of anemia. There is no significant hepatocellular failure in these patients. Although many clinicians think that the frequency of variceal bleeding reduces after puberty, but this has not been confirmed.

Gastic varices are common in EHPVO. According to reports, about 70% children at diagnosis have gastric varices. Most of these are gastroesophageal varices while a few are isolated gastric varices (Sarin, 1992; Arora, 1998; Poddar, 2004). Following eradication of esophageal varices, gastric varices become more evident with increase in risk of bleeding (Poddar, 2004; Goncalves, 2000).

Rectal varices are documented in 80-90% of adult EHPVO cases (Misra, 2005). The scanty data in children indicate presence of rectal varices in 36-64% (Heaton, 1993; Yachha, 1996). It also probably related to the severity and duration of portal hypertension or site of obstruction (at the junction of splenic and superior mesenteric veins leading to redistribution of portal pressure along the inferior mesenteric vein) (Misra, 2005; Chawla, 1991; Ganguly, 1995). Appearance of these varices may increase after obliteration of the esophageal varices.

5.2.1.1 Risk factors for bleeding and rebleeding after initial sclerotherapy

Bleeding from varices occurs usually due to erosion or rupture of variceal vessel wall. Bleeding due to erosion of vericeal wall is precipitated by reflux esophagitis, drug ingestion

(NSAIDs), and febrile illness (Yadav, 1993; Arora, 2002; Lilly, 1982). Size of varix, vessel wall thickness and tissue support also determine the chance of variceal bleeding. Considerable agreement exists regarding the relationship of variceal size to the risk of bleeding. Large variceal size appears to predict bleeding (Rector, 1985). Incomplete variceal obliteration has also been suggested as risk factor for rebleeding (Kokawa, 1993). Vessel wall thickness and tissue support are difficult to assess by endoscopy, but reddish-blue tense varices that are not obliterated on insufflations and congestive mucosa on and around the varices (cherry red spots) are likely to bleed (Alvarez, 1983). Evidence relating to risk of variceal hemorrhage secondary to raised portal pressure is inconclusive.

Our group at AIIMS, New Delhi followed 58 children with EHPVO (age group: 5 months-158 months) who underwent endoscopic sclerotherapy (EST) for a median period of 20.5 months (17-31 months). About half of the patients (28 children) had one or more bleeding episodes (total 88 bleeding episodes) during the follow up period, out of which 21 patients had minor and 7 patients had major bleeding episodes. Congestive gastropathy was observed in all of these patients. The median time interval of occurrence of the any rebleed after completion of EST was 3.5 months [95% CI = 2-7]. Kaplan Meier Survival Analysis indicated that 50 % of patients [95% CI: 34.9 - 63.5%] had first rebleeding episode by 27 months and most of these patients had recurrence of bleeding within 12 months. The relative risks of rebleeding due to risk factors were 2.37 (95% CI = 1.36 - 3.85), 8.9 (95% CI = 2.4 - 23) and 6.1 (95% CI = 3.3 - 10.4) for fever alone, NSAID drug (Ibuprofen and Paracetamol) intake alone and when both fever and drug ingestion respectively. There was no significant difference in the nutritional status of these patients at the end of this follow up period (Arora, 2000).

5.2.2 Mass abdomen

About 10% of the children present with isolated abdominal mass due to splenomegaly (Arora, 1998; Mittal, 1994). EHPVO is associated with splenomagaly and size of spleen usually increases with age and it may even reach the right iliac fossa. Massive splenomegaly may result in anemia and thrombocytopenia due to hypersplenism in about 1/3rd of cases. In cases of acute variceal bleeding, the spleen size may reduce temporarily and reappear on hemodynamic stabilization.

5.2.3 Pain abdomen

Dull abdominal pain may be there due to the splenmegaly. Presence of continuous abdominal pain may indicate splenic infarction or extension of venous thrombosis (Yachha, 1996).

5.2.4 Ascites and edema

Ascites may develop in a proportion of children following hemorrhage or surgery, and are often transient. Ascites have been reported in up to one fifth of children with EHPVO (Webb, 1979; Rangari, 2003). Development of ascites signifies and circulatory changes. Some patients may also have pedal edema. Some children with EHPVO develop intractable ascites with no evidence of hepatic dysfunction. These patients are likely to benefit from large peritoneal drainage or may require shunt surgery. In all cases of ascites, hepatic dysfunction must be carefully looked for.

5.2.5 Ectopic varices

These have been reported in 27-40% of patients with EHPVO, and are commonly seen in the duodenum, anorectal region and gallbladder bed (Sarin, 2006). Bleeding from the varices in duodenum and anorectal regions are not uncommon.

5.2.6 Jaundice

Jaundice is rarely a presenting feature of EHPVO and is generally due to portal biliopathy or stricture of bile duct in longstanding cases.

5.3 Complications and sequelae of EHPVO

EHPVO is associated with several complications and sequalae those need mention from the clinical manifestation and management point of views. The documented sequelae observed in long course of EHPVO are as follows.

5.3.1 Portal biliopathy

Portal biliopathy refers to abnormalities of the extrahepatic and intrahepatic bile ducts in patients with portal hypertension. These include compression by paracholedochal collaterals on bile ducts resulting in displacement, narrowing, strictures, angulation, dilatations and irregularity of bile ducts. Extrinsic compression, ischemia, and a combination of both have been proposed as the possible mechanisms for this. Although portal biliopathy features have been reported in 80-100% of adult patients with EHPVO on endoscopic retrograde cholangio-pancreatography (ERCP), up to one fifth are symptomatic (Dilawari, 1992; Khuroo, 1993; Malkan, 1999; Nagi, 2000; Poddar, 2001). These changes may become severe enough to cause obstructive jaundice and choledocholithiasis and cholelithiasis due to bile stasis. Cholangiographic changes are also evident in children with EHPVO, but mostly symptomatic in adulthood (Poddar, 2011). Although, biliary abnormalities are common in portal hypertension, only a few patients present with jaundice, pain and cholangitis. Choleodocholithiasis has been reported to occur in 17% of patients with portal biliopathy (Bhatia, 1995). ERCP is the definitive method for diagnosis of biliopathy. MRCP is a good non-invasive alternative to ERCP. However, as the majority of patients with biliopathy are asymptomatic, ERCP is recommended only if a therapeutic intervention is contemplated.

5.3.2 Ectopic varices

Gall bladder varices are observed in 34% of adult patients with EHPVO (Chawla, 1995). Reports in children with EHPVO are scanty. Presence of portal vein thrombosis is an important determinant for the development of gall bladder varices. Rectal varices may be seen in up to 80% of patients with EHPVO and the development is related to the duration. These varices may also bleed profusely (Sarin, 1992). Gall bladder varices are reported in 12-30% of adults with EHPVO (Chawla, 1995; West, 1991).

5.3.3 Gastropathy and colopathy

Gastropathy and colopathy represent congested mucosa at different parts of gastrointestinal tract which may present as occult gastrointestinal bleeding, but sometimes also as overt bleeding. About one fourth of the EHPVO children have gastropathy at presentation, but the prevalence increases significantly (2 times or more) after variceal eradication (Hyams, 1993; Poddar, 2004). Portal colopathy may be seen in up to half of the patients with EHPVO (Sarin, 1992; Arora, 1999).

5.3.4 Hyersplenism

Massive splenomegaly may cause pooling and excessive destruction of the pooled blood cell components leading to thrombocytopenia, leucopenia and anemia. It can also predispose to infection and or bleeding. The hypersplenism does not correlate with splenic size. Splenic sequestration crisis may occur leading to hypovolemic shock and death.

6. Specific issues in children

6.1 Growth retardation

EHPVO in children often reported to be associated with growth retardation.

Reports from India indicated that the majority of the Indian children with EHPVO were stunted compared to the national control or to the National Center for Health Statistics (USA) reference (Mehrotra, 1997; Sarin, 2002; Arora, 2000). It also appears that the lean mass building is more likely to be affected than the fat storage (Mehrotra, 1997). Although the growth velocity have not been documented in any of these studies but the Z scores for height and weight at diagnosis and during follow-up after sclerotherapy were not statistically different. One study from India reported lower growth velocity in majority of children with EHPVO compared to the controls despite adequate nutrition (Sarin, 1992). A report from Brazil (n= 24; median age 5.9 years) reported that children with EHPVO had adequate growth for the age at diagnosis and over follow up period of 3.8±2.5 years compared to the NCHS reference (Bellomo-Brandao, 2003). Although the exact mechanism of the growth failure is not known, the following possible mechanisms have been proposed.

- Poor substrate utilization or/and malabsorption due to portal hypertensive enteropathy is the proposed mechanism. This is supported by improved growth in many children with EHPVO after shunt surgery (Menon, 2005).
- Impaired synthesis of growth factors due to shunting of blood away from the liver is another hypothesis . Significantly increased levels of growth hormone and decreased levels of insulin-like growth factor-1 (IGF-1) and insulin-like growth factor binding protein-3 (IGFBP-3) have been noted in EHPVO patients, suggesting growth hormone resistance (Mehrotra, 1997; Nihal, 2009). It is proposed that reduced portal blood flow results in decreased insulin reaching the liver and thereby decreased production of IGF-I and IGFBP-3. Shunt surgery, mesenterico-left portal vein bypass (MLPVB) with improvement in growth parameters in children with EHPVO supports this hypothesis (Lautz, 2009; Stringer, 2007).
- Frequency of bleeding has been linked to the growth in these children. It is observed that children with frequent bleeding have severe growth retardation while children with asymptomatic course are normal or near normal (Mowat, 1987).

While growth parameters in children with EHPVO have shown improvement after shunt surgery, no change in growth trend were documented in children after sclerotherapy (Arora, 2000; Sarin, 2002), even with adequate caloric intake (Sarin, 1992). This also support the proposed substrate metabolism, insulin and growth factor mediated mechanisms as the cause of growth failure. The overall nutritional status and underlying etiology and the associated complications of recurrent bleeds may influence the growth in children with EHPVO.

6.2 Mental function and encephalopathy

Mild cognitive and psychomotor deficit has been reported in patients with EHPVO in absence of liver disease (Sarin, 2006). Hyperammonia as a result of porto-systemic shunting in EHPVO may lead to generalized low grade cerebral edema. Abnormal cognitive functions may be evident on neuropsychological tests in some of these patients with apparently normal neurological status, which is described as having minimal hepatic encephalopathy. Normal liver functions probably reduce the severity of hepatic encephalopathy. A term type B hepatic encephalopathy has been proposed for this condition (Ferenci, 1998). In a recent Indian series of children, about one-third of children with EHPVO had abnormal neuropsychological test findings (visual-motor coordination and spatial orientation), raised blood ammonia, abnormal MRI signal, and abnormal brain metabolites on MR spectroscopy compared to the normal children (Yadav, 2010).

7. Diagnosis and investigation findings

A child with upper gastrointestinal bleeding (manifesting as either hematemesis and/or malena) and splenomegaly but no features of chronic liver disease is likely to be suffering from EHPVO. Normal liver function test and absence of virologic markers in a child with portal hypertension further suggest towards EHPVO. But the other causes of non-cirrhotic portal hypertension and compensated childhood cirrhosis are to be excluded. Imaging of spleno-portal axis is the mainstay for the diagnosis of EHPVO. According to Baveno V consensus statement, EHPVO is diagnosed by Doppler US, CT, or MRI, which demonstrate portal vein obstruction, presence of intraluminal material or portal vein cavernoma. Recent EHPVO is characterized by demonstrated portal venous obstruction without cavernoma (De Franchis, 2010).

7.1 Ultrasonography

Ultrasound (US) is a reliable non-invasive diagnostic tool with a high degree of accuracy for the detection of blockage in splenoportal axis and portal portal cavernoma, and is the investigation of choice (Sharma, 1997). Usually the normal portal vein and branches are invisible and are replaced by multiple tortuous collateral veins with hepatopetal flow, the cavernomatous transformation of the portal vein. Large collateral vein may simulate to be portal vein but tortuosity and presence of surrounding small channels help in differentiation. Portal vein thrombus may be observed as an echogenic lesion within the vessel, although a recently formed thrombus may be anechoic. Colour Doppler imaging is very helpful in detecting portal vein flow and diagnosing portal vein obstruction, spleno-portal collaterals and shunts with sensitivity of 70 - 90% and specificity of 99% (Nyandak, 2011). Ultrasound may also indicate about the liver pathology (size and echogenicity) and portal biliopathy which may have intrahepatic bile duct dilatation due to compression of the common bile duct by the cavernoma. Endoscopic ultrasound (EUS) may further advance the diagnostic accuracy in patients with portal vein thrombosis.

7.2 CECT

In contrast-enhanced CT scan, thrombus may be seen as a nonenhanced intraluminal-filling defect. CECT has the advantage of displaying varices and parenchymal hepatic abnormalities also. The combination of CT scan and Doppler ultrasound is common in the evaluation of portal vein obstruction.

7.3 MRI

MRI and magnetic resonance angiography (MRA) are helpful for evaluating hepatic parenchymal details, to quantitate portal and hepatic vessel flow for planning of interventions, such as shunt surgery. MRI can help detecting and differentiating acute and old clots and blockage due to tumor thrombi. MRI and MRA are highly sensitive and specific for detecting both the thrombi and submucosal, serosal, paraoesophageal collaterals. CT and MRA may be more useful for detecting the recent EHPVO.

7.4 Endoscopy

Upper gastrointestinal endoscopy is must for all EHPVO patients to detect the status of varices, any site of bleeding and associated congestive gastropathy. For detecting the lower gastrointestinal bleeding due to rectal or colonic varices, lower gastrointestinal endoscopy may be needed.

7.5 Biochemical tests

Biochemical liver function test parameters are usually within normal range, unless associated with underlying liver disease. But with longstanding disease liver function may deteriorate. Viral markers for hepatotropic viruses are to be screened as these children are at high risk for blood borne transmission due to repeated blood transfusions. Liver biopsy is not indicated in EHPVO unless underlying liver pathology is suspected. Screening for prothrombotic disorders may help in identifying underlying coagulopathy.

7.6 Radionuclide scan

In cases of gastrointestinal bleeding not visualized by endoscopy may need radionuclide scanning (99m Technetium sulfur colloid and 99m technetium pertechnate labeled RBCs) to detect the site of bleeding if not evident on endoscopy. 99m Tc scan can even detect bleeding rate of 0.1-0.5 mL/min. Radionuclide scan is only rarely required.

7.7 Additional tests

Additional tests like ERCP and MRCP may be indicated to detect the presence of portal biliopathy, if suspected. Endoscopic retrograde cholangiopancreatography (ERCP) is indicated for confirming portal biliopathy, particularly if there are features of cholangitis or obstructive jaundice.

8. Management

8.1 Concepts and principles of management

Management of EHPVO depends on the age of the patient, the site of obstruction and the clinical presentation. Liver involvement necessitates modification in approach to management. Management in children also needs to address the nutrition to ensure optimal growth.

8.2 Prophylaxis

Prophylaxis is very important in cases with portal hypertension to reduce the risk of initial bleeding (primary prophylaxis) or rebleeding (secondary prophylaxis) through reducing the vascular pressure in splenoportal axis.

8.2.1 Primary prophylaxis

Evidence on the role of primary prophylaxis in the management of portal hypertension and portal hypertension has not been adequately studied in children. Use of Propranolol (1-2mg/kg body weight/day) as primary prophylaxis has been shown to be effective in reducing bleeding compared to secondary prophylaxis (15.6% vs 53.3% respectively) (Ozsoylu, 2000). So, children with varices on endoscopy are to be initiated on beta blocker, but follow up endoscopy is to be done to check the status every 6-12 monthly interval.

Prophylactic endoscopic sclerotherapy and variceal obliteration is also in practice. Use of prophylactic EST children with portal hypertension had lower bleeding episodes (24%) compared to controls (42%) over a median follow-up of 4.5 years (Goncalves, 2000). But the evidence and experience in children is limited to support recommendation of prophylactic EST or EVL.

8.2.2 Secondary prophylaxis

Evidences on secondary prophylaxis are better than that of primary prophylaxis. Beta blockers are in use for reducing portal pressure and thereby reducing risk or variceal bleeding. Propranolol is commonly used at dosage 2mg/kg body weight/day in 2 divided doses. Heart rate is monitored and dosage is adjusted to prevent fall of heart rate more than 20% of baseline or absolute heart rate below 60/minute. Metaanalysis indicated the benefit of beta blocker in reducing variceal bleeding (Sarin, 1996). About 20% of the patients do not respond to the beta blockers and some cannot be given due to contraindications like congestive heart failures, peripheral vascular diseases, chronic obstructive pulmonary diseases, asthma, and insulin dependent diabetes mellitus.

8.2.3 Management of gastrointestinal bleeding

Gastrointestinal bleeding related to portal hypertension and EHPVO may be of variceal or mucosal in nature. Variceal bleeding may be of acute nature presenting as life threatening episode or of chronic with recurrent episodes or malena with or without anemia. Usually acute variceal bleedings are life threatening with sudden onset and may be associated with loss of large volumes of blood. It can be fatal in 30-40% of cases.

Quick history and clinical examination is to be done to rule out non-GI bleeding, assess the severity of bleeding and hemodynamic status. There is no controversy about the management of acute variceal bleeding and involves the following five steps.

i. Emergency resuscitation and hemodynamic stabilisation
ii. Identification of source and site of bleeding
iii. Stopping bleeding source
iv. Monitoring
v. Variceal obliteration

While planning the management of acute bleeding, along with hemodynamic status, liver function status is also to be assessed as soon as possible to plan the management strategy. Urgent upper gastrointestinal endoscopy should be undertaken at the earliest after full resuscitation, to identify source and to intervene to stop bleeding.

8.3 Endoscopic management of variceal bleeding

8.3.1 Management of esophageal variceal bleeding

Endoscopic variceal sclerotherapy (EST) and endoscopic variceal ligation (EVL) are two effective methods of controlling acute bleeding from esophageal varices. EST involved injection of sclerosant (sclerotherapy) into the varix and/or surrounding submucosa. Commonly used sclerosants ate sodium morruhate (1.5%), tetradecyl sulfate (0.5-1%), phenol (3%) and polidocanol (1%). EST is effective in eradicating esophageal varices in 88-100% cases. However, complications like retrosternal pain (30-60%), fever (39%), ulcer (8% to 30%) and stricture (6% to 20%) are often encountered with EST (Poddar, 2011; Arora, 2002). Meta-analysis of sclerotherapy in adults has demonstrated its advantage over vasopressin; and comparable efficacy with somatostatin or octreotide in controlling acute variceal bleeding (De Franchis, 1999). On the other hand endoscopic variceal ligation (EVL) involves ligation of the varix using bands. Although, EVL has the advantages of rapid eradication of varices requiring fewer sessions and portending fewer complications, use in younger children (< 2 years) may be an issue. Over the years, EVL has become the preferred mode of treatment of variceal bleeding in adults. However, the additional cost of banding is a constraint, especially in developing countries. The limited experience of EVL in children suggests its superiority over EST (Zargar, 2002).

Newer endoscopic treatment modalities like thermal coagulation, electrocoagulation and laser photocoagulation are also being tried in adults. But the experience in children is not available.

After initial control of bleeding, eradication of varices is necessary to prevent subsequent bleeding. Either EST or EVL in isolation or EST followed by EVL can be adopted for this. EVL alone although appears to be simpler and effective for initial eradication of varices, recurrence of varices is high, as obliteration of smaller varices and perforators is difficult. EST/EVL sessions are repeated at 1-2 weekly interval and usually 6-10 sessions are required to completely obliterate the esophageal varices. Variceal recurrence has been documented in 40% of children after 2 years of EVL (McKiernan, 2002). So a combination of EVL and EST, initial EVL followed by low-dose EST appears to be more effective in children. It reduces the sessions required, complications associated with large-dose EST for initial variceal eradication and the risk of variceal recurrence. Two studies from India supported this combination intervention (Poddar, 2005; Poddar, 2011).

8.3.2 Management of gastric varices

The experience in children is limited. Gastric varices bleed less frequently but when they do, they bleed profusely. Endoscopic injection of tissue adhesive agent (n-butyl 2 cyanoacrylate) has been effective in controlling such bleeding, as EST or EVL may not be suitable. Large gastric varices with or without bleeding are considered as an indication for shunt surgery.

8.3.3 Management of colorectal varices

Management of bleeding rectal varices include sclerotherapy or band ligation. For presence of larger rectal varices and colopathy with or without bleeding, shunt surgery may be considered.

8.4 Medical management of variceal bleeding

Several drugs are also used to reduce the portal venous pressure and thereby variceal bleeding before undertaking endoscopic therapy. These agents enable stabilization of the patient till the definite interventions are done or if not possible.

8.4.1 Vasopressin

Vasopressin is the most potent splanchnic vasoconstrictor. It reduces blood flow to all splanchnic organs, decreasing portal venous inflow and thereby decreasing portal pressure. Vasopressin is administered as continuous infusion and increased till maximum dosage is reached in titration with the bleeding. The infusion is to be continued for at least 24-48 hours after stoppage of bleeding. In about 60% of the patients bleeding is controlled using this agent (Tuggle, 1988). Although this drug in adults has been shown to control bleeding yet the mortality does not decrease and dose at highest level may be associated with complications. The usage is limited by adverse effects related to vasoconstriction in splanchnic bed leading to bowel ischemia and systemic circulation resulting in hypertension and myocardial ischemia. To minimize the systemic adverse effects, vasopressin should always be accompanied by intravenous nitroglycerin.

8.4.2 Terlipressin

Terlipressin is a synthetic analogue of vasopressin with longer biological activity and significantly fewer adverse effects. Terlipressin may have more sustained hemodynamic effects in patients with bleeding varices.

8.4.3 Somatostatin

Natural hormone somatostatin decreases portal pressure by causing splanchnic vasoconstriction. It is associated with lesser side effects compared to vasopressin. There is limited experience in children. In adult patients somatostatin is effective in 64-92% cases (Burroughs, 1990). Blood sugar is to be monitored every 6 hourly to detect hypoglycemia.

8.4.4 Octreotide

It is a synthetic analogue of somatostatin and effective in controlling acute variceal bleeding in most (84-95%) of adult patients. It can be given as infusion or intermittent subcutaneous injections. Monitoring is similar to Somatostatin.

There are limited data on the use of pharmacological agents for the control of acute bleeding in children with EHPVO. However, if EHPVO is due to acute thrombophilia, there is a theoretical risk of a decrease in splanchnic blood flow induced by bleeding and by therapeutic vasconstrictive agents that may cause extension of thrombus in the portal venous system resulting in intestinal ischemia.

8.5 Other interventions to manage acute variceal bleeding

8.5.1 Balloon tamponade

Direct compression of varices with balloon (Sengstaken-Blackemore tube) has been used to stop bleeding. The smaller tube is also available for pediatric use. It has two balloons, one each for esophageal and gastric compression and one lumen for aspiration of gastric contents. The balloons are inflated using air or saline to compresses the varices at gastroesophageal junction and in esophagus. Intermittent deflation of the balloon is important to prevent mucosal ischemia. Aspiration is another complication that can potentially be fatal. This balloon device can control acute variceal bleeding up to 80% of cases (Pitcher, 1971; Brodoff, 1980). Positioning of the tube and is to be confirmed with plain X-ray abdomen. Selection of appropriate tube size, experience and following simple precautions are necessary to prevent tissue necrosis and aspiration.

8.5.2 Transjugular Intrahepatic Portosystemic Shunt (TIPS)

This procedure involves creation of an artificial shunt between hepatic vein and portal vein within liver via a catheter passed through internal jugular vein. The tract maintained by a self expandable metal stent enables decompression of the portal system. Mostly it has been used in patients of cirrhosis awaiting liver transplantation. This is a technically difficult procedure, costly and needs expertise. The experience in children is small and success rates variable between 75-90% (Heyman, 1999).

8.5.3 Management of mucosal bleeding

Bleeding or oozing may occur from mucosal lesions associated with congestive gastropathy or colopathy due to portal hypertension. Management of gastropathy involves neutralization of the gastric acid and stoppage of bleeding from the sites/ lesions. The medications used are:

- Antacids for neutralizing the gastric acid.
- H_2 receptor blockers or proton pump blockers to reduce the gastric acid secretion. Duration of use is to be decided based on the nature of mucosal lesion.

- Sucralfate forms a protective barrier on the mucosal lesions and prevent contact of gastric acid.

Management of colopathy is difficult and the endoscopic photocoagulation or laser coagulation like measures may be helpful. Additionally the beta-blockers are recommended for these patients. Recurrent bleeding from portal hypertensive gastropathy and/or colopathy usually indicates shunt surgery.

The flow chart of managing a child with variceal and/or mucosal bleeding is given below.

Step I

Check and rule out
1. Non-GI bleeding (nasal, respiratory)
2. Red coloring agents

Examine and assess
1. Pulse/BP; Airway/ Breathing status; Cyanosis/ Cold peripheries; Mental status; Jaundice/ Liver size & features of liver failure; Spleen/Ascites

Step II

Assess severity

Moderate	**Severe**	**Very severe**
Malena and/or small bloody gastric aspirate **And** No anemia (Hb >10g/dl) **Or** No orthostatic hypotension **Or** No signs of impaired consciousness	Large bloody gastric aspirate **Or** H/o severe hematemesis **And** Anemia (Hb ≤10g/dl) **Or** Orthostatic hypotension **Or** Tachycardia **Or** Impaired consciousness	Continuing severe hematemesis **And** Hypotension/acidosis/altered sensorium **Or** Severe anemia (Hb ≤7g/dl) **Or** Signs of heart failure **Or** Signs of other organ dysfunction
↓	↓	↓

Step III

Observation/ Hospitalize	**Hospitalize**	**Hospitalize in ICU**

Observation/ Hospitalize:

1. Initial assessment
1.1 CBC, PT, PTT, electrolytes

Hospitalize / Hospitalize in ICU:

1. Immediate action
1.1. Secure vascular access, central venous access if possible
1.2. Oxygen inhalation
1.3. Prepare for blood tansfusion
1.4. Nasogastric aspiration, urinary catheterization
1.5. Get CBC, PTT, PT. electrolyte done
1.6. Monitor hematocrit 2-3 hrly till bleeding stops and then 4-6 hrly
1.7. Mechanical ventilation if needed

2. Treat hypovolemia
2.1 Fluid bolus (normal saline/ Ringers lactate 20-30ml/kg)
2.2 Repeat as necessary while monitoring the BP, pulse, CVP, urine output and hematocrit (maintain at 30%)

3. Improving oxygenation
3.1 Blood transfusion (whole blood if available till bleeding stop and then packed cells)
3.2 Adjust oxygen and ventilation settings

4. Correcting coagulation problem (if present)
4.1 Administer FFP/ platelets if needed

Step IV

Observation/ Hospitalize:

2. Determine bleeding site
2.1 Diagnostic endoscopy
2.2 Additional investigation to detect the bleeding site (as necessary)

Hospitalize / Hospitalize in ICU:

5. Determine bleeding site
5.1 Emergency endoscopy after initial stabilization
5.2 Additional investigation to detect the bleeding site (as necessary)

Bleeding site(s)

Variceal bleed	**Mucosal lesion**	**Bleeding source not known**

Step V	Bleeding site(s)		
	Variceal bleed	**Mucosal lesion**	**Bleeding source not known**
	Management of variceal bleed	**Management of mucosal bleed**	**Management if source is not known**
	1. Emergency EST/ EVL If patient is hemodynamically stable. **2. Pharmacological therapy** If patient is hemodynamically unstable or facilities of emergency endoscopic therapy are not available. The following options are used. **2.1 Vassopressin** - Start with 0.1 U/min IVdiluted in 2 ml/kg of 5% dextrose infusion and increase by 0.05U/min hourly to a maximum dosage according to age (0.2U/min if <5 yrs, 0.3U/min if 5-12 yrs and 0.4 U/min if >12 yrs) - continue drug for 24-48 hrs after stoppage of bleeding - Taper gradually 0.1-0.2U/min every 4 hrs - Monitor cardiac rate and rhythm - Watch for peripheral ischemia **2.1.1 Nitroglycerine** - Always start with vasopressin at 0.25-0.5µg/kg/min IV - Taper gradually with Vassopressin **2.2 Terlipressin** - 2 mg every four hourly IV till bleeding free interval of 24-48 hours **2.3. Somatostatin** - 250 µg bolus followed by 250µg/hr as continuous infusion. - Monitor blood sugar 6 hourly **2.4. Octreotide** - 1-2 µg/kg bolus (maximum 50 µg) followed by 0.4-2µg/kg/hr (maximum 50 µg/hr) as continuous infusion - Monitor blood sugar 6 hourly	**1. Reducing gastric acid secretion** **1.1 H2 blockers** - Ranitidine 2 mg/kg/dose twice a day orally/ IV daily **1.2 Proton pump blockers** - Omeprazole 10 mg orally twice a day (< 3 years) or 20 mg orally twice a day (> 3 years) **1.3 Coating the lesions** - Sucralfate 500 mg oraly four times a day **2. Continue Propranolol** **3. Treating underlying factors** - Omission of offending drugs - Manage coagulation disorders, DIC - Management of sepsis, if associated	**1.Identifying site of bleed** - Radionuclide scan - Capsule endoscopy, if possible **2. Manage like mucosal bleeds** - Till site identified and definite management is done/available **3. Treat the underlying factors**

Flow chart: Evaluation and management of upper gastrointestinal bleeding

8.5.4 Management of acute portal thrombosis

Spontaneous resolution of recent portal thrombus is rare. Management includes conservative medical and surgical interventions. The symptomatic patients with recent EHPVO should be started on low molecular weight heparin immediately after detection followed by oral anticoagulant therapy. In asymptomatic patients, if detected early, anticoagulation should be considered. Dosage of anticoagulation therapy is to be titrated with target to maintain international normalized ration (INR) around 2-3. Baveno V consensus statement recommends anticoagulation for at least three months, unless long term/lifelong therapy is indicated for underlying persistent prothrombotic state (De Franchis, 2010). Repeat Doppler is to be done after 3-6 months to check for recanalisation of portal vein. In acute thrombosis cases, evidence of infection must be ruled out. If any evidence of infection is there, antibiotic therapy should be given. Advanced minimally invasive intervention techniques like direct thrombolysis of portal vein, thrombolysis through TIPS are being used. But experience in children is limited.

8.5.5 Surgical management of EHPVO

Surgical management of EHPVO includes shunt and non-shunt procedures. The shunt procedures aim at reducing portal pressure by diverting the blood from the high-pressure portal venous system to the systemic circuit. Shunt surgeries are recommended for EHPVO cases not responding to medical and endoscopic management and if associated with complications. The indications for shunt surgery include failure of endotherapy to control bleeding, presence of gastric or ectopic varices (not amenable to endoscopic management), and associated complications like portal biliopathy and large rectal varices. Emergency shunt surgery is undertaken now only rarely due to wide availability of endoscopic management. The additional indications for shunt surgery include portal biliopathy, severe growth failure, massive splenomegaly, hypersplenism, rare blood group, isolated splenic vein thrombosis, non- compliance of elective EST/EVL and poor chance of follow up (living in remote area). Individualization of each child with EHPVO for shunt surgery is to be done considering all the aspects and in consultation with the surgical team.

Shunts may be non-selective shunts or selective shunts, partial shunts and the more recently introduced "Rex shunt"(mesenterico-left portal bypass).

The non-selective shunts enable complete decompression of the entire portal venous system by diverting total portal blood flow away from the liver. These shunts are end to side and side-to-side portacaval shunts, central lienorenal shunt, end to side mesocaval shunt and large diameter interposition portacaval or mesocaval shunts. Although these shunts are effective in controlling variceal bleeding, encephalopathy is a concern in patients with poor liver functions. Follow up studies have shown shunt patency in 85-98% of children with long term survival in >95% cases (Lautz, 2009; Bismuth, 1980; Alvarez, 1983; Gauthier, 1989; Mitra, 1993; Prasad, 1994; Orloff, 1994; Superina, 2006; Shariff, 2010). Risk of variceal recurrence and re-bleed is there in case of shunt blockage. But there is no report of post shunt encephalopathy in EHPVO cases. Splenectomy usually done with central lienorenal shunt has not been found to be associated with an increased risk of post-splenectomy sepsis (Arora, 2002).

The selective shunts divert the blood of gastroesophageal-splenic segment and maintain the blood flow in mesenteric segment based on the functional classification of portal venous system into the splenogastric and mesenteric segments. This enables portal decompression with maintenance of hepatopetal portal perfusion, mesenteric venuos pressure and hepatotrophic factors. Distal splenorenal shunt, a selective shunt has technical advantage of lower chance of post-shunt encephalopathy. The mesoportal bypass (MPB) is a recent advancement in shunt restoring mesenteric blood flow to the liver through the Rex venous recessus (interposition of a jugular venous allograft between the superior mesenteric vein and the intrahepatic left portal vein). This "Rex shunt" restores the physiological hepatopetal flow and thereby corrects the liver dysfunction, coagulation parameters and also improves the growth potential (Superina, 2006; Mack, 2003; Lautz, 2009). It appears that doing the Rex shunt early after diagnosis rather than waiting till complications will be beneficial. But in want of clear evidence and experience, there is no consensus on this issue.

A subgroup of EHPVO patients may not be suitable for shunt surgery in view of complicated vascular anatomy due to extensive thrombosis of the splenoportal axis, prior splenectomy or a previously performed but failed shunt procedure. These cases merit non-surgical management and non-shunt surgical procedures, if required.

8.5.6 Portosystemic shunt vs endoscopic sclerotherapy

In a randomized clinical trial by our group in India, we assessed the complications, technical problems and rebleeding rates after EST and shunt surgery. Out of the 297 children with EHPVO screened, 156 children were randomized into surgical and EST groups (78 children in each group). Out of the 78 children randomized into in surgical group, 8 opted out before intervention and 28 could not undergo surgery due to technical reason (blockage of splenic vein) and hence received EST. Out of the 78 children in EST group, 75 children undergone EST (2 opted out before intervention and 1 died). The children were followed up (median follow up period 24 months; range: 21-29 months). The pooled incidence of bleeds decreased from 0.11/month in pre-intervention period to 0.014/month in post-intervention phase, when both the interventions were considered together. The fall in the incidence rate for major bleeds was higher (0.05 to 0.002) than that for minor bleeds (0.06 to 0.013). Survival analysis showed that among the children who underwent EST, 25% had rebleeding by 16.9 months after intervention while 50% had rebleeding by 38.4 months. Children who underwent surgery had rebleeding by 18.3 months in 25% subjects and less than half of these subjects ever rebled. Survivor function at various 6 monthly time intervals during follow up was similar between EST and surgery groups. This was true for any kind of re-bleed; major bleeds and minor bleeds. Relative risk of rebleeding after controlling for period of follow up was similar for all types of bleeds. Recurrence of esophageal varices was higher in surgery group compared to the EST group. By 6 months, half of the patients who underwent surgical intervention, had recurrence of varices, while the same was observed after 24 months in patients who underwent EST. But the risk of rebleeding was not influenced by recurrence of varices. Risk of re-bleeding was associated with the age of intervention, lesser rebleeding was noticed among children aged >10 years. Hypersplenism was observed in 17 children in the EST group compared to 3 children in the surgery group. Eight patients in the EST group died compared to 6 patients in the surgery group. It appeared from this data that both EST and surgery appear to perform equally well to control rebleeding in EHPVO patients. (Arora, 2004).

8.6 Management of special situations related to EHPVO

8.6.1 Portal biliopathy

Symptomatic portal biliopathy is a definite indication for intervention. Primary biliary tract surgery is associated with significant morbidity and mortality due to presence of extensive collaterals around the bile ducts. Some experts suggest shunt surgery first and if it fails to resolve biliary obstruction, then to undertake staged biliary surgery (Chaudhary 1998). While others recommend endoscopic management of biliary obstruction first and if obstruction persists, then to do the shunt surgery (Khare, 2005). Presence of choledocholithiasis without biliary stricture can be managed by endoscopic sphincterotomy and stone removal. Presence of stricture may need balloon dilatation and stent placement. In cases of endoscopic failure, portosystemic shunt followed by biliary surgery should be undertaken (Khare 2005). There is no clear consensus regarding timing of biliary surgery after shunt surgery. The experience in children in this context is limited. Children with portal biliopathy undergoing shunt surgery may have normalization of serum aminotransferases and gamma glutamyl transpeptidase (GGT) levels within 1 to 6 weeks after surgery (Gauthier, 2005). Shunt surgery is indicated in children with symptomatic portal biliopathy or even asymptomatic portal biliopathy in presence of growth failure, symptomatic hypersplenism or ectopic varices.

8.6.2 Hypersplenism

Traditionally, hypersplenism has been treated by splenectomy, open or laparoscopic. In view of the risk of overwhelming sepsis in children who are asplenic, the risks and benefits must be carefully weighed when splenectomy is being considered. Age of removal of spleen is an important consideration; risk of overwhelming sepsis may increase if child is less than 5 years. Vaccines against pneumococcus, *Haemophilus influenza and* meningococcus should be administered to all children particularly these below 5 years, who are about to undergo splenectomy, at least 10 days before splenectomy. Additionally, antibiotic prophylaxis (penicillin) is recommended to asplenic children who have not received vaccines. In recent times, alternative technique of partial splenic embolisation (PSE) is in use (Dwivedi, 2002). It causes ischemic necrosis of a part of spleen and thereby decreases in splenic size and hypersplenism. It allows the preservation of adequate splenic tissue and thereby prevents the immunological function and protection against overwhelming infection.

8.6.3 Coagulopathy

The management of coagulopathy depends on the cause. There is no consensus or clear guideline about anticoagulant therapy for prothrombotic conditions in chronic EHPVO. In a patient with established chronic EHPVO, anticoagulants are recommended only if there is a history of recurrent thrombotic episodes and after shunt surgery (Valla, 2002). Anticoagulation therapy is contraindicated in cases with active variceal bleeding and can be initiated after variceal obliteration and patient is on beta blocker drug.

9. Natural history

The natural course of EHPVO is mainly determined by the age at presentation, presence or absence of underlying liver disease, associated systemic diseases. Most patients with EHPVO in the absence of liver disease and systemic disease have a relatively benign course. Morbidity is mainly related to variceal bleeding, recurrent thrombosis (if associated with prothrombotic disorder), symptomatic portal biliopathy, and hypersplenism. In case of children with EHPVO, especially in developing countries, nutritional status and growth retardation also influence the outcome.

9.1 Quality of life with EHPVO

Children with EHPVO suffering in view of repeated episodes of bleeding, undergoing diagnostic and therapeutic procedures, associated complications and morbidities, delayed growth, may have psychological issues that may impeded their ability and potential in physical, emotional, social, academic and other extracurricular segments. A study among

Indian children with EHPVO compared the quality of life (QOL) scores in children before variceal eradication, after variceal eradication and after surgery with controls. Overall children with EHPVO had lower median QOL scores in physical, emotional, social, and school functioning health domains compared to controls. Esophageal variceal eradication had no significant effect on QOL, but QOL improved after surgery. Most likely surgery provided a feeling of cure and reduced further risk and morbidity for both patient and the parents and thus resulted improvement in psychological status. Spleen size significantly influenced quality of life (QOL) scores and children with massive splenomegaly had poor QOL scores as compared with patients with mild and moderate splenomegaly. Total, physical, and psychosocial QOL scores were significantly lower in children with growth retardation. Both spleen size and growth retardation were independent predictors that affect the QOL (Radha Krishna, 2010).

10. Prognosis

Unlike patients with chronic liver disease, patients with EHPVO have a good prognosis as their liver functions are preserved. Mortality is mainly due to variceal bleeding and it is to the tune of 5% (Mowat, 1986). Long term studies after endotherapy have shown almost no mortality. Many of these bleeding episodes occurred within the first 4-10 years of variceal eradication (Zargar, 2004; Thomas, 2009; Stringer, 1994). The risk of rebleeding reduces with increasing age, especially after 10 years of age. With increasing age of survival, children with EHPVO are likely to face the longer term consequences in nutrition, mental function and portal biliopathy. Long term follow up studies shall be able to answer some of the unanswered issues in EHPVO.

11. Conclusion

Extrahepatic portal venous obstruction is the commonest cause of portal hypertension and variceal bleeding in children. With the availability of diagnostic facilities and effective endotherapy, the mortality due to EHPVO related emergencies has become rare. But with increasing survival, the sequelae and related morbidities are rising. The evolving surgical interventions have raised the hope of averting the long term complications of EHPVO. Further generation of evidence on etiology and course of disease including the effect of management in children with EHPVO is required, especially in developing countries. At the same time availability of trained manpower and facilities for management of acute emergencies and advanced surgical interventions will further improve the outcome.

12. References

[1] Alvarez F, Bernard O, Brunell F, Hadchouel P, Odièvre M, Alagille D. Portal obstruction in children. II. Results of surgical portosystemic shunts. *J Pediatr*. 1983;103:703–7.

[2] Alvarez F, Bernard O, Brunnelle F et al. portal hypertension in children: Clinical investigations and hemorrhage risk. *J Pediatr* 1983; 103: 696-702.

[3] Arora NK, Ganguly S, Mathur P, Ahuja A, Patwari A. Upper Gastrointestinal bleeding: Etiology and Management. *Indian J Pediatrics*. 2002; 69:155-168.

[4] Arora NK, Lodha R, Gulati S, Gupta AK, Mathur P, Joshi MS, et al. Portal hypertension in north Indian children. *Indian J Pediatr*. 1998;65:585–91.

[5] Arora NK. (Principal Investigator), Mathur P, Das MK.. Project titled "Risk factors for re-bleeding after endoscopic sclerotherapy in children with Extrahepatic Portal Hypertension" . Funded by Indian Council of Medical Research (ICMR). India, Report 2000. Conducted at All India Institute of Medical Sciences, New Delhi.

[6] Arora NK. (Principal Investigator), Jain S, Mathur P, Das MK. Project titled "Management of Extra-hepatic Portal Hypertension in Childhood: Efficacy and Efficiency of Endoscopic Sclerotherapy versus Porto-systemic Shunt Surgery". Funded by Indian Council of Medical Research (ICMR). India, Report 2004. Conducted at All India Institute of Medical Sciences, New Delhi.

[7] Bellomo-Brandão MA, Morcillo AM, Hessel G, Cardoso SR, Servidoni MFPC, da-Costa-Pinto EA. Growth assessment in children with extra-hepatic portal vein obstruction and portal hypertension. *Gastroenterologia Pediatrica.*2003; 40:247-250.

[8] Bhatia V, Jain AK, Sarin SK. Choledocholithiasis associated with portal bililopathy in patients with extrahepatic portal vein obstruction and management with endoscopic sphincterotomy. *Gastrointest Endosc* 1995;42:178-181.

[9] Bhattacharya M, Makhani G, Kannan M, Ahmed R P, Gupta P K, Saxena R. Inherited prothrombotic defects in Budd-Chiari syndrome and portal vein thrombosis: a study from North India. *Am J Clin Pathol* 2004; 121: 844-7.

[10] Bismuth H, Franco D, Alagille D. Portal diversion for portal hypertension in children. The first ninety patients. *Ann Surg*. 1980; 192:18–24.

[11] Brodoff M, Conn HO. Esophageal tamponade in the management of bleeding esophageal varices. *Dig Dis Sc*. 1980; 25: 267-272.

[12] Burroughs AK, McCormick PA, Hughes MD et al. Randomized double blind placebo controlled trial of somatostatin for variceal bleeding. Emergency control and prevention of early variceal bleeding. *Gastroenterology* 1990; 99: 1388-1395.

[13] Chaudhary A, Dhar P, Sarin SK, Sachdev A, Agarwal AK, Vij JC, et al. Bile duct obstruction due to portal biliopathy in extrahepatic portal hypertension: surgical management. Br J Surg. 1998; 85: 326–9.

[14] Chawla A, Dewan R, Sarin SK. The fequency and influence of gall bladder varices on gall bladder function in patients with portal hyper tention . *Am j Gastroenterol* 1995;90:2011-14

[15] Chawla Y, Dilawari JB. Anorectal varices—their frequency in cirrhotic and non-cirrhotic portal hypertension. *Gut.*1991; 32: 309–11.

[16] De Franchis R, On behalf of the Baveno V Faculty. Revising consensus in portal hypertension: Report of the Baveno V consensus workshop on methodology of diagnosis and therapy in portal hypertension. *Journal of Hepatology* 2010; 53: 762–768.

[17] De Franchis R, Primignani M. Endoscopic treatment for portal hypertension. *Seminars in Liver Disease* 1999; 19: 499-455.

[18] Dilawari JB, Chawla YK. Pseudosclerosing cholangitis in extrahepatic portal venous obstruction. *Gut*. 1992; 33: 272–6.

[19] Dilawari JB, Ganguly S, Chawla Y. Non-cirrhotic portal fibrosis. *Ind J Gastroenterol* 1992; 11: 31-36.

[20] Dubuisson C, Boyer-Neumann C, Wolf M, Meyer D, Bernard O. Protein C, protein S and antithrombin III in children with portal vein obstruction. *J Hepatol*. 1997; 27: 132–5.

[21] Dwivedi MK, Pal RK, Dewanga L, Nag P. Efficacy of partial splenic embolisation in the management of hypersplenism. *Indian J Radiol Imaging*. 2002;12:371-4

[22] Ferenci P, Lockwood A, Mullen K, et al. Hepatic Encephalopathy: Definition, Nomenclature, Diagnosis, and Quantification: Final Report of the Working Party at the 11th World Congress of Gastroenterology, Vienna, 1998. *Hepatology* 2002; 35: 716-21.
[23] Ganguly S, Sarin SK, Bhatia V, Lahoti D. The prevalence and spectrum of colonic lesions in patients with cirrhosis and noncirrhotic portal hypertension. *Hepatology*. 1995; 21: 1226–31.
[24] Gauthier F, De Dreuzy O, Valayer J, Montupet P. H-type shunt with an autologous venous graft for treatment of portal hypertension in children. *J Pediatr Surg*. 1989; 24: 1041–3.
[25] Gauthier-Villars M, Franchi S, Gauthier F, Fabre M, Pariente D, Bernard O. Cholestasis in children with portal vein obstruction. *J Pediatr*. 2005; 146: 568–73.
[26] Goncalves ME, Cardoso SR, Maksoud JG. Prophylactic sclerotherapy in children with esophageal varices: long-term results of a controlled prospective randomized trial. *J Pediatr Surg*. 2000; 35: 401–5.
[27] Heaton ND, Davenport M, Howard ER. Incidence of haemorrhoids and anorectal varices in children with portal hypertension. *Br J Surg*. 1993;80:616–8.
[28] Heyman'MB, LaBerge JM. Role of transjugular intrahepatic portosystemic shunt in the treatment of portal hypertension in pediatric patients. *J Pediatr Gastroenterol Nutr* 1999; 29 : 209-249.
[29] Hyams JS, Treem WR. Portal hypertensive gastropathy in children. *J Pediatr Gastroenterol Nutr*. 1993;17:13–8.
[30] Khare R, Sikora SS, Srikanth G, Choudhuri G, Saraswat VA, Kumar A, et al. Extrahepatic portal venous obstruction and obstructive jaundice: approach to management. *J Gastroenterol Hepatol*. 2005;20:56–61.
[31] Khuroo MS, Yattoo GN, Zargar SA, Javid G, Dar MY, Khan BA, et al. Biliary abnormalities associated with extrahepatic portal venous obstruction. *Hepatology*. 1993;17:807–13.
[32] Kokawa H, Shijo H, Kubara K, et al. Long term risk factors for bleeding after first course of endoscopic injection sclerotherapy : A univariate and multivariate analysis. *Am J Gastroenterol* 1993; 88 : 1206 - 1211.
[33] Koshy A, Bhasin DK, Kapoor KK. Bleeding in extrahepatic portal vein obstruction. *Indian J Gastroenterol*. 1984;3:13–4.
[34] Larroche J. Umbilical catheterization: its complications. *Biol.Neonate* 1970;16:101-103.
[35] Lautz TB, Sundaram SS, Whitington PF, Keys L, Superina RA. Growth impairment in children with extrahepatic portal vein obstruction is improved by mesenterico-left portal vein bypass. *J Pediatr Surg*. 2009;44:2067–70.
[36] Lilly JR, Stiegmann GV, Stellin G. Esophageal endosclerosis in children with portal vein thrombosis. *J Pediatr Surg* 1982;17:571-575.31.
[37] Mack CL, Superina RA, Whitington PF. Surgical restoration of portal flow corrects procoagulant and anticoagulant deficiencies associated with extrahepatic portal vein thrombosis. *J Pediatr*. 2003;142:197–9.
[38] Malkan GH, Bhatia SJ, Bashir K, Khemani R, Abraham P, Gandhi MS, et al. Cholangiopathy associated with portal hypertension: diagnostic evaluation and clinical implications. *Gastrointest Endosc*. 1999;49:344–8.
[39] McKiernan PJ, Beath SV, Davison SM. A prospective study of endoscopic esophageal variceal ligation using multiband ligator. *J Pediatr Gastroenterol Nutr*. 2002;34:207–11.

[40] Mehrotra RN, Batia V, Dabadghao P, Yachha SK. Extrahepatic portal vein obstruction in children: anthropometry, growth hormone, and insulin-like growth factor I. *J Pediatr Gastroenterol Nutr* 1997;25:520-3.

[41] Menon P, Rao KL, Bhattacharya A, Thapa BR, Chowdhary SK, Mahajan JK, et al. Extrahepatic portal hypertension: quality of life and somatic growth after surgery. *Eur J Pediatr Surg*. 2005;15:82–7.

[42] Misra SP, Dwivedi M, Misra V, Dharmani S, Kunwar BK, Arora JS. Colonic changes in patients with cirrhosis and in patients with extrahepatic portal vein obstruction. *Endoscopy*. 2005;37:454–9.

[43] Mitra SK, Rao KLN, Narasimhan KL, Dilawari JB, Batra YK, Chawla Y, et al. Side-to-side lienorenal shunt without splenectomy in noncirrhotic portal hypertension in children. *J Pediatr Surg*. 1993;28:398–401; discussion 401–2.

[44] Mittal SK, Kalra KK, Aggarwal V. Diagnostic upper GI endoscopy for hematemesis in children: experience from a pediatric gastroenterology centre in north India. *Indian J Pediatr*.1994;61:651–4.

[45] Mowat AP. Disorders of portal and hepatic venous systems. In: Mowat AP, editor. Liver disorders in childhood. 2nd ed. London: Butterworths; 1987.p.298-323.

[46] Mowat AP. Prevention of variceal bleeding. *J Pediatr Gastroenterol Nutr*. 1986;5:679–87.

[47] Nagi B, Kochhar R, Bhasin D, Singh K. Cholangiopathy in extrahepatic portal venous obstruction. Radiological appearances. *Acta Radiol*. 2000;41:612–5.

[48] Nihal N, Bapat MR, Rathi P, Shah NS, Karvat A, Abraham P, et al. Relation of insulin-like growth factor-1 and insulin-like growth factor binding protein-3 levels to growth retardation in extrahepatic portal vein obstruction. *Hepatol Int*. 2009;3:305–9.

[49] Nyandak T, Prakash P, Das U, Yadav P, Sharma SC, Srivastava D, Rewari BB. Portal Vein Thrombosis - Clinical Profile. *Journal of Indian Academy of Clinical Medicine*. 2011; 12:134-40.

[50] Odievre M, Pige G, Alagille D. Congenital abnormalities associated with extraheptic portal hypertension. *Arch Dis Child* 1977; 52: 383-5.

[51] Orloff MJ, Orloff MS, Rambotti M. Treatment of bleeding esophagogastric varices due to extrahepatic portal hypertension: results of portal-systemic shunts during 35 years. *J Pediatr Surg*. 1994;29:142–51; discussion 151–4.

[52] Ozsoylu S, Kocak N, Demir H, Yuce A, Gurakan F, Ozen H. Propranolol for primary and secondary prophylaxis of variceal bleeding in children with cirrhosis. *Turk J Peidtr* 2000; 42 : 31-33.

[53] Pinto R B, Silveira T R, Bandenilli E, Rohsig L. Portal vein thrombosis in children and adolescents: the low prevalence of hereditary thrombophilic disorders. *J Pediatr Surg* 2004; 39: 1356-61.

[54] Pitcher JL. Safety and effectiveness of the modified Sangstaken-Blackemore tube. A prospective study. *Gastroenterology* 1971; 61 : 291-298.

[55] Poddar U, Bhatnagar S, Yachha SK. Endoscopic band ligation followed by sclerotherapy: Is it superior to sclerotherapy in children with extrahepatic portal venous obstruction? *J Gastroenterol Hepatol*. 2011;26:255–9.

[56] Poddar U, Borkar V. Management of extra hepatic portal venous obstruction (EHPVO): current strategies. *Tropical Gastroenterology* 2011;32(2):94–102.

[57] Poddar U, Thapa BR, Bhasin DK, Prasad A, Nagi B, Singh K. Endoscopic retrograde cholangiopancreatography in the management of pancreaticobiliary disorders in children. *J Gastroenterol Hepatol*. 2001;16:927–31.

[58] Poddar U, Thapa BR, Puri P, Girish CS, Vaiphei K, Vasishta RK, et al. Non-cirrhotic portal fibrosis in children. *Indian J Gastroenterol.* 2000;19:12–3.
[59] Poddar U, Thapa BR, Rao KL, Singh K. Etiological spectrum of esphageal varices due to portal hypertension in Indian children: is it different from the West? *J Gastroenterol Hepatol.* 2008;23:1354–7.
[60] Poddar U, Thapa BR, Singh K. Band ligation plus sclerotherapy versus sclerotherapy alone in children with extrahepatic portal vein obstruction. *J Clin Gastroenterol.* 2005;39:626–9.
[61] Poddar U, Thapa BR, Singh K. Endoscopic sclerotherapy in children: experience with 257 cases of extrahepatic portal venous obstruction. *Gastrointest Endosc.* 2003;57:683–6.
[62] Poddar U, Thapa BR, Singh K. Frequency of gastropathy and gastric varices in children with extrahepatic portal venous obstruction treated with sclerotherapy. *J Gastroenterol Hepatol.* 2004;19:1253–6.
[63] Prasad AS, Gupta S, Kohli V, Pande GK, Sahni P, Nundy S. Proximal splenorenal shunts for extrahepatic portal venous obstruction in children. *Ann Surg.* 1994;219:193–6.
[64] Radha Krishna Y, Yachha SK, Srivastava A, Negi D, Lal R, Poddar U. Quality of Life in Children Managed for Extrahepatic Portal Venous Obstruction. *J Pediatr Gastroenterol Nutr.* 2010;50: 531–536
[65] Rangari M, Gupta R, Jain M, Malhotra V, Sarin S K. Hepatic dysfunction in patients with extrahepatic portal venous obstruction. *Liver Int* 2003 Dec; 23: 434-9.
[66] Rector WG, Reynolds TB. Risk factors for hemorrhage from esophageal varices and acute gastric erosions. *Clin Gastroenterol.* 1985;14:139-153.
[67] Sarin SK, Agarwal SR. Extrahepatic portal vein obstruction. *Semin liver disease.* 2002; 22:43-58.
[68] Sarin SK, Bansal A,Sasan S ,et al. Portal vein obstruction in children leads to growth retardation. *Hepatology* 1992;15:229-233.
[69] Sarin SK, Guptan RC, Jain A, Sundaram KR. A randomized controlled trial of endoscopic variceal band ligation for primary prophylaxis of variceal bleeding. *Eur J Gastroenterol Hepatol.* 1996; 8 : 337-342.
[70] Sarin SK, Lahoti D, Saxena SP, Murthy NS, Makwana UK. Prevalence, classification and natural history of gastric varices: a long-term follow up study in 568 portal hypertension patients. *Hepatology.* 1992;16:1343–9.
[71] Sarin SK, Sollano JD, Chawla YK, et al on behalf of Members of the APASL Working Party on Portal Hypertension. Consensus on Extra-hepatic Portal Vein Obstruction. *Liver International.* 2006; 26:512-519.
[72] Sharif K, Mckiernan P, de Ville de Goyet J. Mesoportal bypass for extrahepatic portal vein obstruction in children: close to cure for most! *J Pediatr Surg.* 2010;45:272–6.
[73] Sharma MP. Sonographic signs in portal hypertension: a multivariate analysis.*Ultrasound in Medicine & Biology.* 1997; 23: S17-S17.
[74] Sharma S, Kumar SI, Poddar U, Yachha SK, Aggarwal R. Factor V Leiden and prothrombin gene G20210A mutations are uncommon in portal vein thrombosis in India. *Indian J Gastroenterol.* 2006;25:236–9.
[75] Stringer M D, Heaton N D, Karani J., et al. Patterns of portal vein occlusion and their etiological significance. *Br J Surg* 1994; 81: 1328-31.

[76] Stringer MD, Howard ER. Long term outcome after injection sclerotherapy for esophageal varices in children with extra hepatic portal hypertension. *Gut.* 1994;35;257–9.
[77] Stringer MD. Improved body mass index after mesenterico-portal bypass. *Pediatr Surg Int.* 2007;23:539–43.
[78] Superina R, Bambini DA, Lokar J, Rigsby C, Whittington PF. Correction of extrahepatic portal vein thrombosis by the meserteric to left portal vein bypass. *Ann Surg.* 2006;243:515–21.
[79] Thomas V, Jose T, Kumar S. Natural history of bleeding after esophageal variceal eradication in patients with extrahepatic portal venous obstruction; a 20-year follow-up. *Indian J Gastroenterol.*2009;28:206–11.
[80] Thompson EN, Sherlock S.The etiology of portal vein thrombosis with particular reference to the role of infection and exchange transfusion. *Q J Med* 1964;33:465-480.
[81] Tuggle DW, Bennett KG, Scott J, Tunell WP. Intravenous vasopressin and gastrointestinal hemorrhage in children. *J Pediatr Surg* 1988; 23 : 627-629. Bottom of Form
[82] Valla D C, Condat B, Lebrec D. Spectrum of portal vein thrombosis in the West. *J Gastroenterol Hepatol* 2002; 17 (Suppl. 3): S224-7.
[83] Webb L J, Sherlock S. The etiology, presentation and natural history of extra-hepatic portal venous obstruction. *Q J Med* 1979; 192: 627-39.
[84] West MS, Garra BS, Horti SC, et al. Gallbladder varices: Imaging findings in patients with portal hypertension. *Radiology* 1991;179:179-82
[85] Yachha S K, Khandur A, Sharma B C, Kumar M. Gastrointestinal bleeding in children. *J Gastroenterol Hepatol* 1996; 11: 903-7.
[86] Yachha SK, Dhiman RK, Gupta R, Ghoshal UC. Endosonographic evaluation of the rectum in children with extrahepatic portal venous obstruction. *J Pediatr Gastroenterol Nutr.* 1996; 23:438–41.
[87] Yadav S, Dutta A K, Sarin S K. Do umbilical vein catheterization and sepsis lead to portal vein thrombosis? A prospective, clinical and sonographic evaluation. *J Pediatr Gastroenterol Nutr* 1993; 17: 392-6.
[88] Yadav S, Srivastava A, Srivastava A, et al. Encephalopathy assessment in children with extra-hepatic portal vein obstruction with MR, psychometry and critical flicker frequency. *J Hepatology.* 2010; 52 (3): 348-354.)
[89] Zargar SA, Javid G, Khan BA, Yattoo GN, Shah AH, Gulzar GM, et al. Endoscopic ligation compared with sclerotherapy for bleeding esophageal varices in children with extrahepatic portal venous obstruction. *Hepatology.* 2002; 36:666–72.
[90] Zargar SA, Yattoo GN, Javid G, Khan BA, Shah AH, Shah NA, et al. Fifteen-year follow up of endoscopic injection sclerotherapy in children with extrahepatic portal venous obstruction. *J Gastroenterol Hepatol.* 2004; 19:139–45.

4

Portal Vein Thrombosis with Cavernous Transformation in Myeloproliferative Disorders: Review Update

Anca Rosu, Cristian Searpe and Mihai Popescu
University of Medicine and Pharmacy Craiova, Romania

1. Introduction

Portal vein thrombosis (PVT) refers to the complete or partial obstruction of blood flow in the portal vein, due to the presence of a thrombus into the vessel lumen (Bayraktar & Harmanci, 2006)

Cavernous transformation of portal vein consists in the development of a network of tortuous collateral vessels bypassing the obstructive area due to chronic PVT. First described in 1869 by Balfour and Stewart, it was Köbrich in 1928 that used for the first time the term of "cavernoma" to define the newly developed network of small vessels as a result of recanalization of the thrombotic portal vein. Once the liver blood supply decreases significantly, the compensatory mechanism is activated and collaterals begin to form within a few days after the obstruction and organize into a cavernous transformation in 3-5 weeks. (Cai, 2009)

Based on a case previously communicated by us - (A case of portal cavernoma – associated thrombocythemia - A. Rosu, C. Searpe, V. Sbarcea, Z. Stoica, M. Popescu. J Gastrointestin Liver Dis 2007 16(1): 97-100), a review of the published English literature was performed using PubMed® (http://www.ncbi.nlm.nih.gov/PubMed) and Medline database. The search of screened articles was made for the keywords "portal vein thrombosis", "portal cavernoma" and "myeloproliferative disorders" (MPD). Articles were selected if a review of the title and/or abstract suggested the association of portal vein thrombosis with cavernous transformation in patients with myeloproliferative diseases.

2. Epidemiology

2.1 Epidemiology of PVT

In the era of continuous and impressive development of the imagistic techniques (contrast-enhanced ultrasound, spiral CT-scan, high definition MRI etc) the diagnosis of portal vein thrombosis (PVT) is no longer a rare condition since recent studies estimates it's incidence at 1,1% in the general population (Ogren et al., 2006). Also PVT is considered to account for 5 to 10% of patients with portal hypertension (Wang et al., 2005).

The concept of PVT as a rare disease is mainly based on clinical series and case reports (Amitrano, 2004), therefore accurate epidemiological data about PVT are difficult to obtain. An epidemiological study performed and conducted in southern Sweden (Ogren et al., 2006) based on the study of 23 796 autopsies, reported the incidental finding of a PVT in about 1% of the general population. Authors reported that 28% of PVT patients had cirrhosis, 23% primary and 44% secondary hepatobiliary malignancy, 10% major abdominal infectious or inflammatory disease and 3% had a myeloproliferative disorder. Other studies reveal that prevalence of PVT in autopsy studies in USA and Japan ranges from 0.05% to 0.5% (Wang et al., 2005).

Actually, thanks to the availability of more sensitive and less invasive imaging, together with the existence of curative or palliative procedures, PVT is routinely investigated and defined without any difficulty. Thus, PVT seems more frequent than expected: it is estimated to be responsible for 5%-10% of the overall cases of portal hypertension, which can be 40% in western countries (Wang et al., 2005).

2.2 Epidemiology of MPD with PVT

The annual incidence of myeloproliferative syndrome is 2,1-3,5 per 100000 peoples (Kutti & Ridell, 2001). From the four entities comprising the myeloproliferative syndrome according to the FAB classification (essential thrombocythemia, polycythaemia vera, chronic myelogenous leukemia and idiopathic myelofibrosis), essential thrombocythemia is considered the most frequent disease with an annual incidence of 0,7-2,5 per 100000 peoples (Cai et al., 2009; Girodon et al., 2009; Rollison et al., 2008). The transformation to acute myelogenous leukemia is recorded in 0,6-5% of patients and the overall 10-year survival rate is 64-80% (Fenaux et al., 1990).

In many patients with non-cirrhotic non-malignant PVT, a systemic, thrombophilic risk factor is often present. Over the last two decades, some of, either inherited or acquired, systemic conditions that result in a thrombogenic phenotype have been identified as risk factors for the development of PVT.

MPD remains the major latent or patent cause of extrahepatic PVT (Diaz et al., 2001 ; Valla et al., 1988; Valla & Condat, 2000). In non-cirrhotic and non-tumoral PVT cases in the West, MPD (i.e. polycythaemia vera, essential thrombocythaemia and myelofibrosis) with a combination of several prothrombotic factors constitute the most common identifiable cause with an estimated prevalence of 30%-60% (Cai et al., 2009; Kiladjian et al., 2006; Kutti & Ridell, 2001). In another study, a myeloproliferative disorder (MPD) was found in 37% of patients with non-cirrhotic non-malignant PVT (Kiladjian et al., 2006).

Essential thrombocytaemia (ET) is frequently associated with thrombotic complications in the large abdominal vessels. It was reported a prevalence of 4% for abdominal vein thrombosis in 460 consecutive patients with ET (Gangat et al., 2006), but did not provide detailed information on portal vein thrombosis. The risk factors for thrombosis in ET patients include age, thrombotic history, cardiovascular risk factors and genetic or acquired thrombophilia (Landolfi et al., 2008). It seems likely that elevated platelet count is involved in thrombotic events in ET. However, the degree of elevation does not appear to be important, relatively low platelet counts often being associated with thrombosis (Harrison, 2005).

3. Etiology and pathogenesis

Portal vein thrombosis is the result of a complex mechanism involving multiple local and systemic risk factors with effect on coagulability, blood flow and endothelium integrity. Blood flow obstruction in the portal vein is the result of invasion, thrombosis, constriction and frequently, a combination of the above-mentioned mechanisms. A list of most common conditions associated with portal vein thrombosis is presented in table 1 and 2 (Chawla et al., 2009; Gurakan et al., 2004; Hoekstra & Janssen, 2009; Janssen, 2001; Rosendaal, 1999; Valla & Condat, 2000; Valla et al., 2002).

<table>
<tr><td>Inherited</td><td colspan="2">Anticoagulant deficiency syndroms (antithrombin-III, protein-C, protein-S)
Mutation involving coagulating factor II (G20210A) or V (G1691)
Plasminogen deficiency
MTHFR homozygote mutation TT677
TAFI (thrombin activatable fibrinolysis inhibitor) gene mutation
Sickle cell disease</td></tr>
<tr><td rowspan="2">Acquired</td><td colspan="2">Myeloproliferative disorders (polycythemia vera, essential thrombocythemia)
Paroxysmal nocturnal hemoglobinuria
Antiphospholipidic syndrome
Hyperhomocisteinemia
Nephrotic syndrome
Estro-progestative medication
Pregnancy</td></tr>
<tr><td>Autoimmune diseases</td><td>Autoimmune hepatitis
Primary biliary cirrhosis
Systemic lupus erythematosus
Rheumatoid arthritis
Wegener disease
Mixed connective tissue disease
Behcet syndrome</td></tr>
</table>

Table 1. Systemic hypercoagulability conditions associated with portal vein thrombosis

Noteworthy are the local factors predisposing to portal location instead of peripheral venous thrombosis in patients with hypercoagulability associated diseases. These factors are: local inflammatory diseases, injury of the portal venous tract, liver cirrhosis and abdominal cancer (table 2).

Although in most cases thrombosis of the portal vein has an identifiable cause, less than 20% are considered to be idiopathic. In children, umbilical vein sepsis and neonatal umbilical vein catheterization are the main causes of portal vein thrombosis. In adults, liver cirrhosis, abdominal malignant tumors and association of different hypercoagulability states explains the vast majority of portal vein thrombosis.

Liver cirrhosis	
Nodular regenerative hyperplasia	
Abdominal malignant neoplasia	Hepatocarcinoma Cholangiocarcinoma Liver metastasis Gallbladder cancer Pancreatic cancer Liver angiosarcoma
Iatrogenic injury of the portal venous tract	Endoscopic sclerotherapy of esophageal varices Alcoolisation/chemoembolisation/radiofrequency ablation of hepatic tumors TIPS / surgical porto-systemic shunt Hepatectomy or liver transplantation Splenectomy Umbilical vein catheterization Colectomy Gastrectomy Hepatobiliary surgery Gastric banding Fundoplication Portography Peritoneal dialysis Islet-cell injection Surgery of the portal tract Endothelial injury due to cytostatics (cisplatin, cyclophosphamide, methotrexate, 5-fluorouracil) or radiation therapy
Local inflammatory diseases	Omphalitis Cholecystitis Cholangitis Appendicitis Diverticulitis Acute or chronic pancreatitis Tuberculous lymphadenitis Inflammatory bowel diseases (Crohn's disease, ulcerative colitis) Hepatic hydatid cyst Pylephlebitis (frequently due to Bacteroides bacteriemia) Liver abscesses Duodenal ulcer Cytomegalovirus hepatitis Schistosomiasis
Choledochal cyst	
Retroperitoneal fibrosis	
Abdominal trauma	

Portal vein malformations	in children with polimalformation
Cardiovascular diseases	Budd-Chiari syndrome Sinusoidal obstruction syndrome Constrictive pericarditis Tricuspid insufficiency Tumour of the right atrium

Table 2. Local conditions associated with high risk of PVT

In patients with liver cirrhosis the incidence of PVT is reported to be between 6 and 17%, with a higher incidence in more advanced stages of the liver disease. The association between liver cirrhosis and hepatocellular carcinoma increases the incidence of PVT over 44%. Additional attention should be paid in cirrhotic patients with underlying prothrombotic condition due to the non-specific decrease in the plasmatic level of coagulation inhibitors even in well-compensated liver cirrhosis. In a recent study it was showed that patients with chronic liver diseases, especially liver cirrhosis, have an increased relative risk of venous thromboembolism, contradicting the classical hypothesis of autoanticoagulation in cirrhotic patients (Søgaard et al., 2009). This procoagulant status was scientifically related to prohemostatic changes of the coagulation factors recorded in chronic liver diseases: elevated levels of factor VIII and von Willebrand factor concomitant with low levels of protein C, protein S, antithrombin-III, plasminogen and ADAMTS-13 (a naturally occurring plasma metalloprotease that limits in vivo functions of von Willebrand factor on platelets).

Hepatocellular carcionoma and pancreatic cancer are the most frequent abdominal malignancies associated with PVT through a compression/invasion/hypercoagulability mechanisms. Hormonal factors might also play a role in this process, especially in men (Bick, 1992).

Primary myeloproliferative diseases (especially polycytemia vera and essential thrombocythemia) are the most often cause of PVT when cirrhosis or cancer is excluded. In a recent study the incidence of myeloproliferative disorders are estimated to be found in 37% of patients with non-cirrhotic/non-malignant PVT (Kiladjian et al., 2006). These diseases are often asymptomatic at the moment of PVT diagnose and therefore a bone marrow biopsy is required. Recently the discovery of the V617F mutation of the Janus kinase 2 (JAK2) in patients with myeloproliferative disorders has been facilitating the diagnosis. JAK2 mutation it has been identified in 95% of patients with polycythemia vera and in 50 to 60% of patients with essential thrombocythemia. Thus, JAK2 mutation it is now recommended by WHO as a major diagnostic criterion for myeloproliferative disorders (Tefferi et al., 2007).

In a study on 74 women with essential thrombocythemia the incidence of thrombosis was 18%, of which major thrombotic episodes were found in 7% (Tefferi et al., 2000). In another retrospective study of 102 patients with myeloproliferative disorders, the rate of thromboembolic complications in patients with polycythemia vera was 16.7%, 13.8% in patients with myelofibrosis and 7.5% in patients with essential thrombocythemia (Brodmann et al., 2000). The cytoreductive therapy with hydroxyurea and supplemental phlebotomy when necessary significantly reduced the risk of thrombosis when compared to control group treated with phlebotomy alone.

The algorithm proposed by AASLD in 2009 for the identification of the PVT etiology is presented in the next table.

1.	Check first for cirrhosis, cancer of the abdominal organs and an inflammatory focus in the abdomen based on initial CT scan and sonography followed by additional procedures, as appropriate
2.	Check for multiple, concurrent risk factors for thrombosis, in all patients without advanced cirrhosis or cancer
3.	Do not rule out a diagnosis of myeloproliferative disease solely on the basis of normal or low peripheral blood cell counts
4.	When coagulation factor levels are decreased, consider low levels of protein C, protein S or antithrombin as a possible consequence of liver dysfunction; consider inherited deficiency when screening of a first-degree relative is positive

Table 3. Algorithm for investigating the cause of PVT (DeLeve et al., 2009)

4. Pathophisiology

Portal vein thrombosis is the main cause of presinusoidal portal hypertension. Frequently the initial placement of the thrombus is in the portal vein trunk but sometimes it is the result of the extension of a thrombus located on the intrahepatic branches of the portal vein or from the splenic vein. According to the location and extension of the thrombus, a grading system was proposed for a better evaluation of the disease prognosis (Naonami et al., 1992).

Grade of PVT	Thrombus description
1	Occlusion of intrahepatic portal vein branches
2	Occlusion of right or left portal vein main branches
3	Partial occlusion of the portal vein trunk
4	Complete occlusion of the portal vein trunk

Table 4. PVT grading system

As a limited form of PVT, the term of "obliterative portal venopathy" was proposed in order to describe the thrombosis of intrahepatic portal vein branches in the absence of liver cirrhosis, inflammation or hepatic neoplasia (Cazals-Hatem et al., 2011).

Within days after the acute thrombosis of the portal vein, a cavernous transformation is taking place as a result of small varices proliferation around the former portal vein concomitant with a recanalisation of the thrombus through a neoangiogenesis process. The result is a spongy, tendril-like convolution of small vessels developed in the area of porta hepatis in order to compensate and by-pass the obstruction of the blood flow. Additionally, the reduced venous blood supply may be compensated by increasing arterial perfusion, which is documented by Doppler ultrasonography.

Chronic portal hypertension and fibroblasts activation inside the cloth leads to the development of a network of tortuous small vessels inside and around the former portal vein acting like a by-pass for the stenotic segment of the portal vein - the so-called portal cavernoma. This process starts from the moment of the acute thrombosis and evolves over the next weeks and months together with the development of porto-portal and portosystemic collaterals until equilibrium is established between prestenotic and poststenotic segment of the portal vein. Moreover, the development of porto-systemic collaterals may lead to a deterioration of the portal encephalopathy.

The natural history of PVT is still unclear, but two possible mechanisms can be involve in the asymptomatic status of the patients: one of them might be the flux augmentation in the hepatic artery as a compensation of the decreased flow in the portal vein; the second one involves the cavernous transformation with fast development of a tortuous network of collateral veins with periportal distribution around biliary ducts, gallbladder, gastric antrum, duodenu and pancreas (Henderson et al., 1992).

PVT and development of a portal cavernoma determines a prehepatic portal hypertension with an elevated blood pressure in the obstructed splanhnic territory with hepatopetal collateral network, condition known as cavernoma (Ohnishi et al., 1984). As a consequence of PVT with cavernous transformation the portal biliopathy can develop (Perlemuter et al., 1996). Another consequence might be a hyperkinetic status with higher cardiac output and lower vascular resistance due to portal obstruction and to portal-systemic collateral circulation (Ohnishi et al., 1984).

5. Clinical features

Clinical presentation always depends on the onset and the extent of the portal thrombosis as well as of the development of collateral circulation.

5.1 Acute PVT

In acute PVT patients can complain of abdominal pain, nausea, vomiting, fever, diarrhoea and haematochezia - symptoms due to intestinal congestion and ischemia. If venous obstruction is not quickly controlled, some severe complications might occur: enteral perforation, septic shock, peritonitis and exitus due to multiorgan failure. The physical examination reveals splenomegaly in almost all cases, whereas ascites is present before the onset of collateral circulation, caused by intestinal venous stasis (Kocher & Himmelmann, 2005; Ponziani et al., 2010).

5.2 Chronic PVT

Usually asymptomatic, the clinical presentation for PVT is almost always hematemesis/melaena due to variceal bleeding. Abdominal pain is not present commonly unless the extension of the PVT into the mesenteric branches causes mesenteric ischemia. An episode of gastrointestinal bleeding is often reported as the first presenting symptom in about 20%-40% of cases (Hoekstra & Janssen 2009), taking into account that in patients with cirrhosis and PVT the risk for variceal bleeding is estimated to be more than 80-120 times higher than in cases without cirrohsis (Condat et al, 2001). Ascites and encephalopathy are rare events and only transient. They are more frequent after an episode of gastrointestinal bleeding or might be associated with renal failure or sepsis especially in older patients (Sobhonslidsuk & Reddy, 2002).

In pylephlebitis patients usually features high fever and chills associated with painful liver at clinical examination.

Physical examination might be completely normal but, sometimes, cholestasis, cholangitis, choledocholithiasis, cholecystitis might occur, configuring the so-called "portal biliopathy".

6. Biologic and imaging studies

Liver laboratory test are usually normal or characteristic for the underlying liver disease. A cholestatic syndrome can develop in PVT associated with portal biliopathy and the ERCP/MRCP frequently reveals a false image of cholangiocarcinoma due to the external compression of the common bile duct by the tortuous vessels of the cavernoma. In case of pylephlebitis blood culture usually reveals *Bacteroides species* and special attention should be paid for the identification of the abdominal origin of the infection.

Beside the eso-gastric varices revealed by the upped digestive endoscopy, other collateral venous circulation can develop in the gallbladder, duodenal, jejunal or rectal walls.

The abdominal ultrasound with Doppler/power-Doppler examination is the investigation of choice in PVT diagnose (sensitivity over 90%). It reveals the presence of the hypo- or hyperechoic material (depending on the age of the thrombus) inside the portal lumen. The examiner must bear in mind that frequently a difficult-to-identify portal vein suggests an old PVT. Additionally, a study from 2009 revealed that portal flow velocity below 15cm/s is an important predictive factor for PVT development (Søgaard et al., 2009).

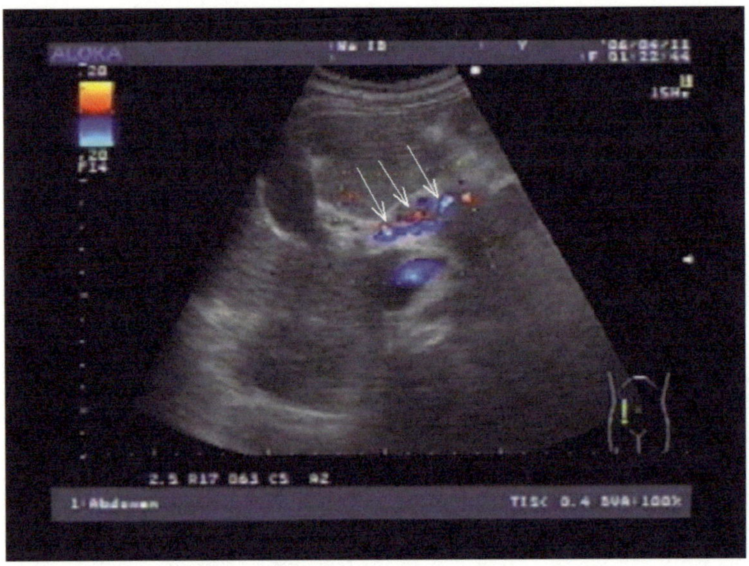

Fig. 1. Patient M.I. 47 years old diagnosed with ET - Doppler ultrasound revealing multiple small venous vessels replacing the former portal vein.

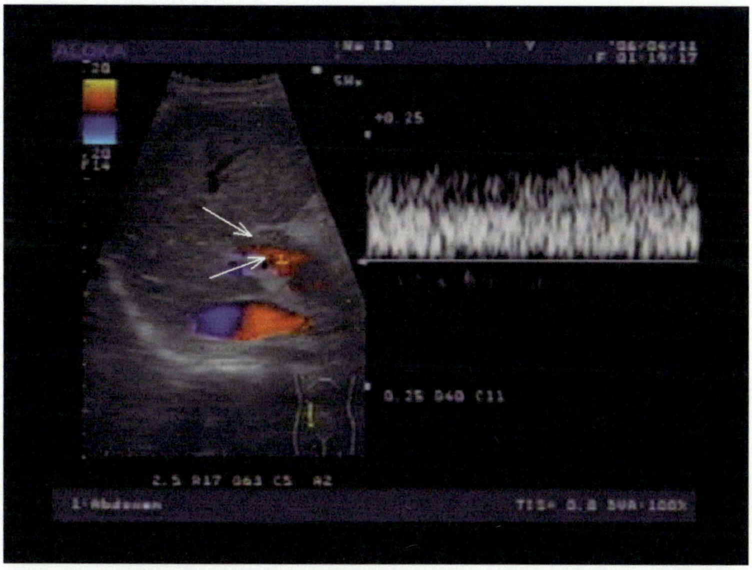

Fig. 2. Patient M.I. - Doppler ultrasound showing an old (hyperechoic) thrombus occluding the portal vein.

The next step in the PVT diagnose algorithm is the magnetic resonance angiography with better results than the CT-scan in identifying the characteristic changes involving the portal trunk.

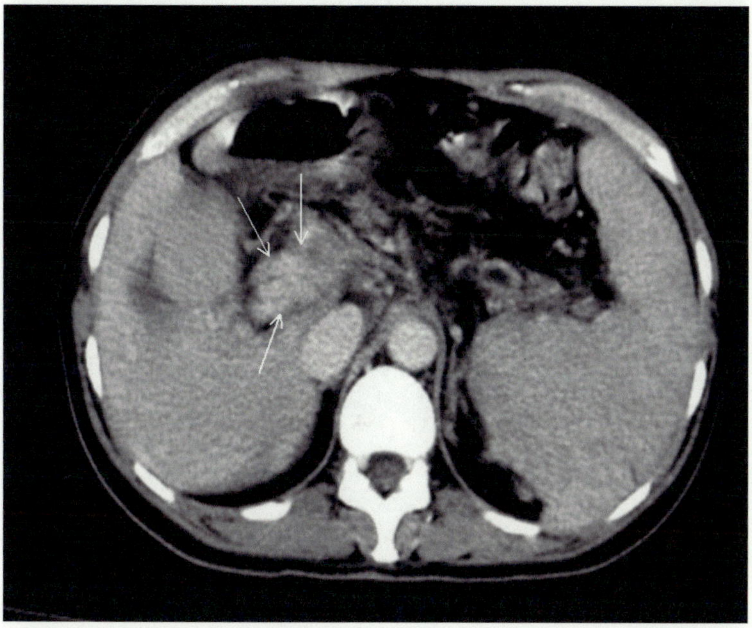

Fig. 3. Patient M.I. - CT scan with i.v. contrast revealing hypodense thrombus and portal cavernoma: heterogonous mass at the level of the portal vein due to cavernouse transformation; homogeneous splenomegaly.

Contrast enhanced ultrasonography is indicated for a better visualization of the thrombus, in differentiating between benign and malignant thrombosis or for the disclosure of cavernous transformation of the portal vein. When differentiating between benign and malignant thrombosis the absence of contrast inside the thrombus is suggestive for benign cloth while contrast enhancement of the thrombus is highly suggestive for neoplastic invasion of the portal vein.

Endoscopic ultrasound was recently added to the imaging armamentory showing a higher sensitivity and specificity than conventional ultrasound and CT/MR-scan in detecting small, non-occlusive thrombi and incipient malignant invasion of the portal and splenic veins.

The portal venography can be useful before surgical treatment is intended. ^{99m}Tc-DTPA (diethylenetriamine pentaacetic acid) scintigraphy reveals only the arterial peak with the absence of the portal peak on the time-activity curve.

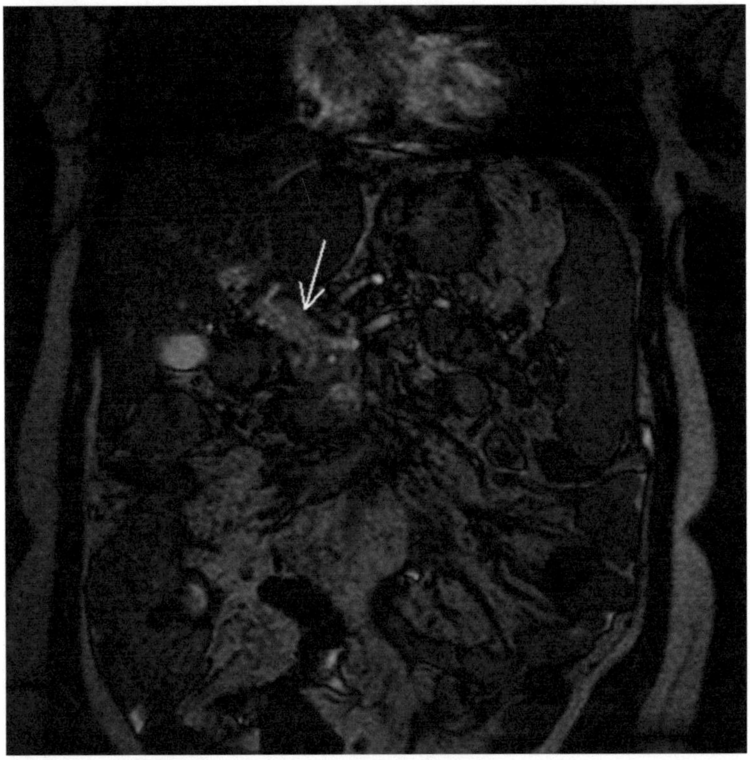

Fig. 4. Patient M.I. - Coronal MRI T2 weighted FRFSE fat-sat depicting portal cavernoma: dilated portal vein with heterogeneous signal due to the cavernous transformation. Associated homogeneous splenomegaly 14 cm diameter.

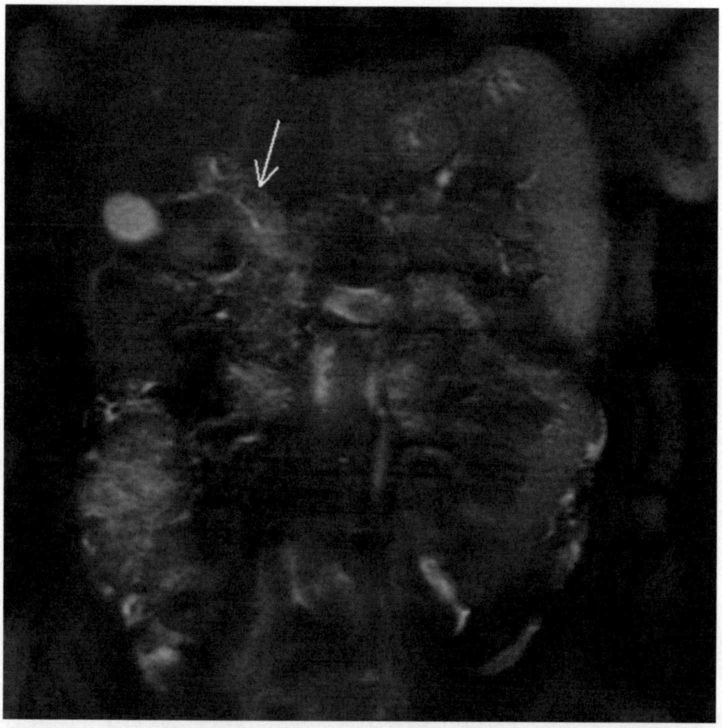

Fig. 5. Coronal MRI T2 weighted fat-sat of the same patient. The permeable lumen having a thread-like hypersignal on T2 weighted image, in the center of the portal vein along with dilated, partially thrombotic, portal vein.

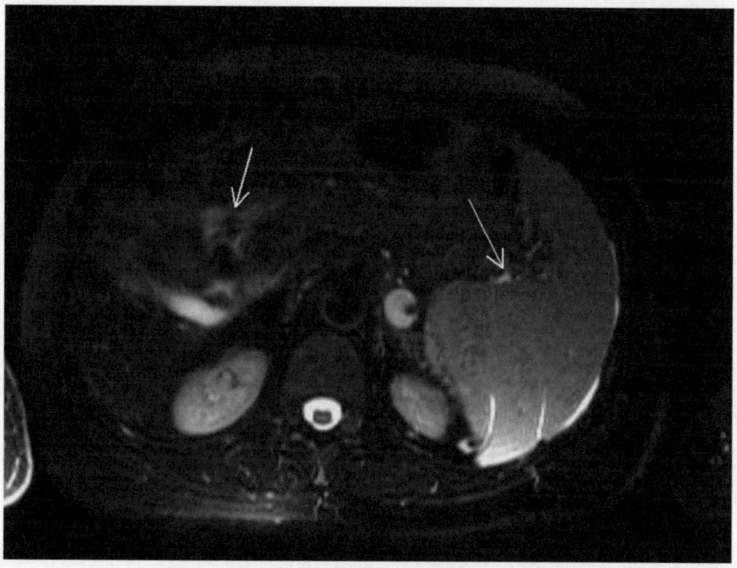

Fig. 6. The same case – axial T2 weighted fat-sat. In addition to the changes of the portal vein the image reveals homogeneous splenomegaly; dilated, partially dilated splenic vein; portal type collateral venous flow.

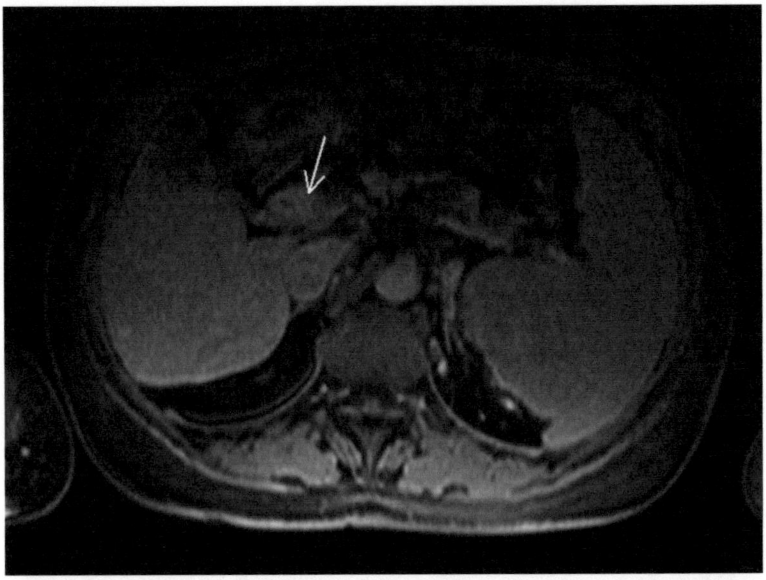

Fig. 7. The same case - axial T1 weighted fat-sat with i.v. contrast. Cavernous transformation of the portal vein with contrast enhancement of the fibrotic thrombi. The central thread-like permeable lumen shows a reduced flow signal.

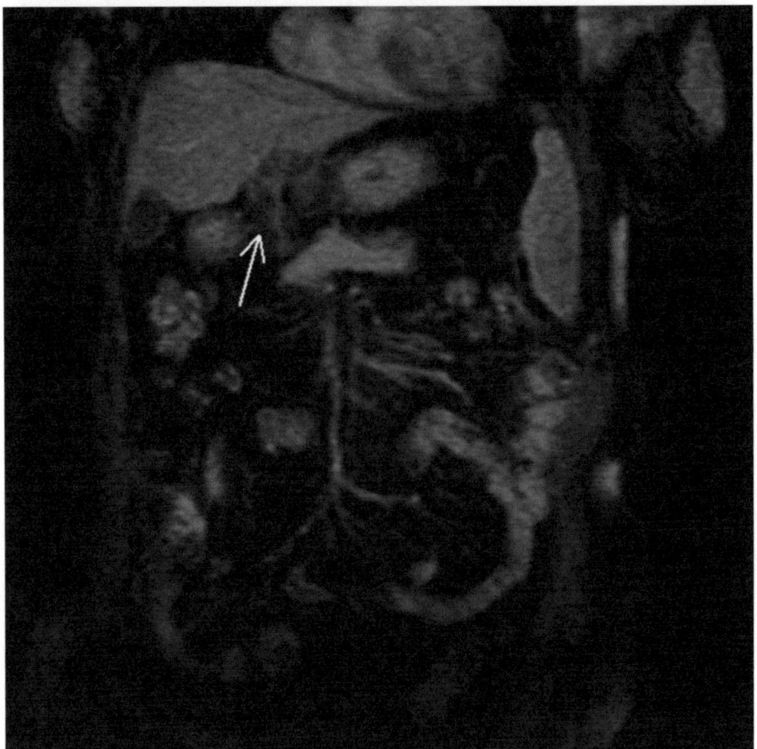

Fig. 8. The same case - coronal T1 weighted fat-sat with contrast. Same changes as in figure 7.

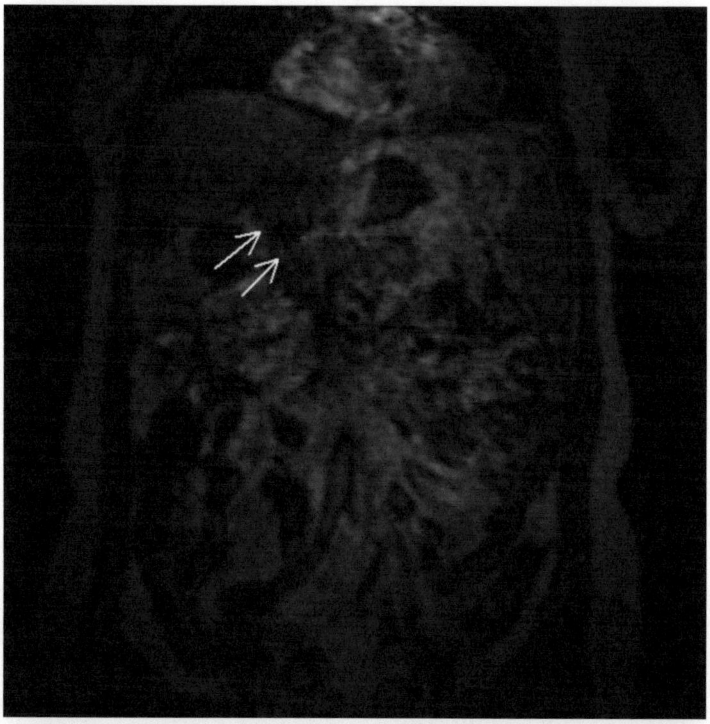

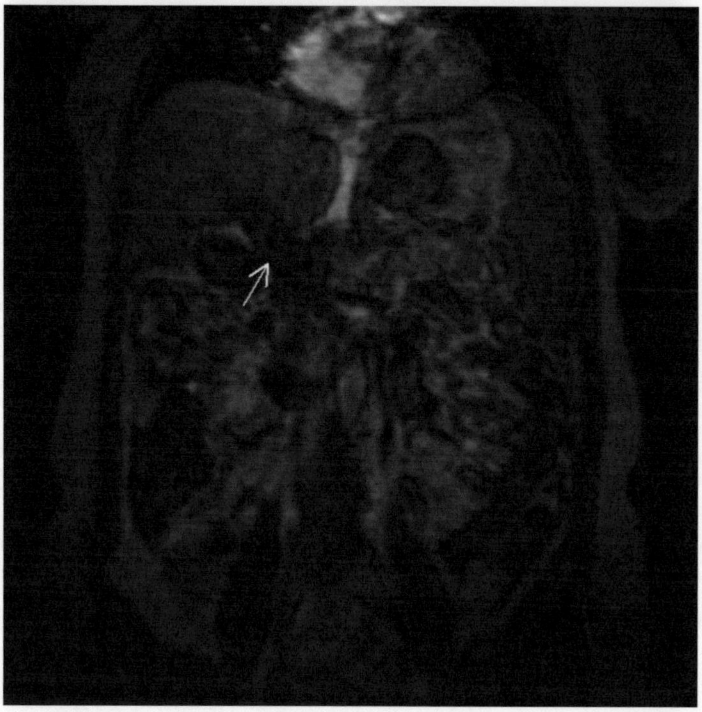

Fig. 9 and 10. The same case – angio-MRI sequence. Inhomogeneous signal of the portal vein with chronic thrombosis.

7. Diagnosis algorithm

The algorithm for PVT diagnose proposed by AASLD in 2009 is presented in the next table.

Acute thrombosis	Chronic thrombosis
1. Consider a diagnosis of acute PVT in any patient with abdominal pain of more than 24 hours duration, whether or not there is also fever or ileus	1. Consider a diagnosis of chronic PVT in any patient with newly diagnosed portal hypertension
2. If acute PVT is suspected, CT scan, before and after injection of vascular contrast agent, should be obtained for early confirmation of diagnosis. If CT scan is not rapidly available, obtain Doppler-sonography	2. Obtain Doppler-sonography, then either CT scan or MRI before and after a vascular contrast agent to make a diagnosis of chronic PVT
3. In patients with acute PVT and high fever and chills, septic pylephlebitis should be considered, whether or not an abdominal source of infection has been identified, and blood cultures should be routinely obtained	3. Base the diagnosis on the absence of a visible normal portal vein and its replacement with serpiginous veins
4. In acute PVT, the possibility of intestinal infarction should be considered from presentation until resolution of pain. The presence of ascites, thinning of the intestinal wall, lack of mucosal enhancement of the thickened intestinal wall,or the development of multiorgan failure indicate that intestinal infarction is likely and surgical exploration should be considered	

Table 5. PVT diagnose algorithm (DeLeve et al., 2009)

8. Treatment

In patients with PVT due to septic conditions (cholangitis, diverticulitis, appendicitis, cholecystitis, umbilical vein infection, pylephlebitis, liver abscesses etc) the prompt initiation of broad-spectrum antibiotic association therapy leads to an efficient repermebilisation of the portal vein within days.

If patient is diagnosed in the recent phase of the PVT (hypoechoic aspect on the ultrasound examination together with blood flow deviation and flux acceleration on Doppler examination) anticoagulant therapy is indicated in order to prevent the total obstruction of the portal vein and the cavernous transformation. Standard heparin or LMWH derivates are initially used followed by oral dicumarinic anticoagulants in order to obtain an INR between 2 and 2,5 with an efficient repermeabilisation in over 80% of cases in the next six months (Valla et al., 2002). As for the peripheral vein thrombosis, the oral anticoagulant therapy is considered to be mandatory for minimum three months and usually is indicated for at least six months. Chronic, indefinite oral anticoagulation is recommended in patients with identified hypercoagulability associated diseases or in presence of thrombus extension into the mesenteric vein.

However, additional concern has been rise over vitamin K antagonists indication in cirrhotic patients due to plasmatic low protein C levels. As protein C is a vitamin K-dependent factor and treatment with vitamin K antagonist may further reduce the plasmatic levels of this anticoagulant protein, the increasing risk for venous thrombosis has been issued. Newly developed direct thrombin inhibitors and inhibitors of activated factor X (e.g. dabigatran, rivaroxaban, apixaban) are considered to be more attractive alternatives to vitamin K antagonists due to their null influence over protein C levels (Franchini & Mannucci, 2009). In addition to their oral administration they have the advantage of not requiring regular laboratory monitoring (such as INR) (Tripodi & Mannucci, 2011).

Concern has been rise also over the safety of chronic anticoagulant therapy in patients with esophageal varices. The few clinical studies addressing this issue (Condat et al., 2001) revealed no significant increase in risk and severity of variceal bleeding.

In initially acute phases, thrombolytic medication (e.g. streptokinase, tPA, alteplase) can be safely initiated especially in patients associating mesenteric ischemia due to thrombus extension in the upper mesenteric vein (Malkowski et al., 2003).

In patients diagnosed with old age thrombus or cavernous transformation of the portal vein the anticoagulant treatment is not indicated due to the lack of efficiency and the associated risk of bleeding.

The major complication of PVT is upper digestive bleeding originating from the eso-gastric varices, with a significant lower mortality rate in patients without liver cirrhosis (aprox. 5%) than in patients with cirrhosis (between 30 and 70%) (Jing-Tong et al., 2005). The endoscopic procedures (band ligation/sclerotherapy) are the first-line treatment indicated in these cases with multiple sessions until the occlusion of the varices. A special attention should be paid when indicating vasoconstrictive agents (e.g. glipresin, terlipresin) due to the possibility of inducind extended intestinal ischemia. Associated oral medication (nonselective beta-blockers +/- long-acting nitrates) prevents the recurrent bleeding. In refractory cases of variceal bleeding and in gastric valices TIPS placement is considered. Malignant portal vein invasion/thrombosis can be safely managed with percutaneous stenting.

More invasive surgical treatment (mesocaval/splenorenal shunts, eso-gastric devascularization) may be necessary in patients with uncontrolled bleeding.

In children it has been recommended the mesenteric-to-left portal vein bypass with very good results in term of rebleeding prevention and improvement of cognitive function.

Initially considered as contraindication for liver transplantation, the complete PVT is now considered to be just a relative contraindication but only in case the superior mesenteric vein is permeable. Partial PVT can be managed by thrombectomy or by-pass techniques.

Portal biliopathy is another potential complication developing in the evolution of PVT with cavernous transformation. It consists in multiple, successive stenosis involving the common bile duct and the hepatic duct as a result of extrinsic compression and/or ischemic fibrosis of the biliary tract. In symptomatic patients (cholangitis, cholecystitis, biliary stones in the CBD, secondary biliary cirrhosis) the portal biliopathy can be addressed with sphincterothomy, stone extraction, stricture dilatation and biliary stanting together with a porto-systemic shunt in order to reduce the external compression of the biliary tract.

From the systemic conditions associated with portal cavernoma, the myeloproliferative syndrome is by far the most frequent one (37% of patients with non-cirrhotic non-malignant PVT) (Kiladjian et al., 2006). To prevent thrombotic complication in chronic myeloproliferative disorders, platelet-lowering agents are used to address the thrombocitemia-associated risk. Hydroxyurea, a ribonucleotide reductase inhibitor with myelosuppressive action, is the first line indication administered on a 500mg PO bid regimen. A platelet-specific lowering agent (Anagrelide) is available on a 0,5mg PO tid regimen for the patients with intoleration to hydroxyurea. For a more efficient myelosuppressive action Interferon-alpha is recommended on a 5MU SC tiw regimen. Despite their leukemogenic action, radiophosphorus (^{32}P) and alkylating agents (e.g. chlorambucil) may be useful as backup regimens in case of recurrent disease (Tefferi et al., 2001). The goal of platelet-lowering medication is to maintain the platelet level under 400000/mm^3 in the high-risk patients (Regev et al., 1997; Storen & Tefferi, 2001). A more aggressive approach like bone marrow transplantation should be considered only in exceptional cases.

9. Prognosis

In the absence of liver cirrhosis and neoplasia the development of portal cavernoma is usually asymptomatic until the first variceal bleeding and has a better prognosis in comparison with variceal bleeding caused by cirrhosis (Janssen et al., 2001).

Except the variceal bleeding, the natural history of portal cavernoma is unremarkable until the development of two other complications: intestinal ischemia (due to extension of the thrombus in the mesenteric vein) and portal biliopathy (common bile duct dilation with cholestatic syndrome).

Although ET usually carries the best prognosis among the MPD, portal vein thrombosis was identified as a risk factor for poor survival, which appears to be the result of increased mortality from acute leukemic or myelofibrotic transformation and hepatic failure (Gangat et al., 2006).

10. References

Amitrano L, Guardascione MA, Brancaccio V, Margaglione M, Manguso F, Iannaccone L, Grandone E, Balzano A. Risk factors and clinical presentation of portal vein thrombosis in patients with liver cirrhosis. *J Hepatol,* 2004;40:736-741

Bayraktar Y, Harmanci O. Etiology and consequences of thrombosis in abdominal vessels. *World J Gastroenterol,* 2006;12:1165-1174

Bick RL. Coagulation abnormalities in malignancy: a review. *Semin Thromb Hemost,* 1992;18:353-372

Brodmann S, Passweg JR, Gratwohl A. et al. Myeloproliferative disorders: complications, survival and causes of death. *Ann Hematol,* 2000;79:312–8

Cai XY, Zhou W, Hong DF, et al. A latent form of essential thrombocythemia presenting as portal cavernoma. *World J Gastroenterol,* 2009;15(42):5368-70

Cazals-Hatem D, Hillaire S, Rudler M et al. Obliterative portal venopathy: portal hypertension is not always present at diagnosis. *J Hepatol,* 2011;54(3):455-61

Chawla Y, Duseja A, Dhiman RK. Review article: the modern management of portal vein thrombosis. *Aliment PharmacolTher,* 2009;30:881-89416

Cohen J, Edelman RR, Chopra S. Portal vein thrombosis: a review. *Am J Med,* 1992;92:173-182

Condat B, Valla D. Nonmalignant portal vein thrombosis in adults. *Nat Clin Pract Gastroenterol Hepatol,* 2006;3(9):505-15

Condat B, Pessione F, Hillaire S, et al: Current outcome of portal vein thrombosis in adults: Risk and benefit of anti-coagulant therapy. *Gastroenterology,* 2001;120:490

De Gaetano AM, Lafortune M, Patriquin H, et al. Cavernous transformation of the portal vein: patterns of intrahepatic and splanchnic collateral circulation detected with Doppler sonography. *AJR Am J Roentgenol,* 1995;165:1151-5

de Suray N, Pranger D, Brenard R. Portal vein thrombosis as the first sign of a primary myeloproliferative disorder: diagnostic interest of the V617F JAK-2 mutation. A report of 2 cases. *Acta Gastroenterol Belg,* 2008;71(1):39-41

DeLeve LD, Valla DC, Garcia-Tsao G. Vascular disorders of the liver. *Hepatology,* 2009;49(5):1729-64

Diaz E, Nahon S, Charachon A et al.Thrombose portale recente regressive sous anticoagulants secondaire a un syndrome myeloprolifferatif latent, une mutation G20210A du gene de la prothrombine et un syndrome des antiphospholipides. *Gastroenterol Clin Biol,* 2001;25:549-551

Dumortier J, Vaillant E, Boillot O, et al. Diagnosis and treatment of biliary obstruction caused by portal cavernoma. *Endoscopy,* 2003;35:446-50

Fenaux P, Simon M, Caulier MT, et al. Clinical course of essential thrombocythemia in 147 cases. *Cancer,* 1990;66(3):549-56

Fimognari FL, Violi F. Portal vein thrombosis in liver cirrhosis. *Intern Emerg Med,* 2008;3(3):213-8

Franchini M, Mannucci PM. A new era of anticoagulants. *Eur J Intern Med,* 2009; 20:562-8

Galati G, Gentilucci UV, Sansoni I, et al. A mocking finding: portal cavernoma mimicking neoplastic mass. First sign of myeloproliferative disorder in a patient with Janus kinase2 V617F mutation. *Eur J Gastroenterol Hepatol,* 2009;21(2):233-6

Gangat N, Wolanskyj AP, Tefferi A. Abdominal vein thrombosis in essential thrombocythemia: prevalence, clinical correlates, and prognostic implications. *Eur Jhaematol,* 2006;77:327-333

Girodon F, Bonicelli G, Schaeffer C, et al. Significant increase in the apparent incidence of essential thrombocythemia related to new WHO diagnostic criteria: a population-based study. *Haematologica,* 2009;94(6):865-9

Gurakan F, Eren M, Kocak N, et al: Extrahepatic portal vein thrombosis in children: Etiology and long-term follow-up. *J Clin Gastroenterol,* 2004;38:368

Harrison CN. Essential thrombocythaemia: challenges and evidence-based management. *Br J Haematol,* 2005;130:153-165

Henderson JM, Gilmore GT, Mackay GJ et al. Hemodynamics during liver transplantation: the interaction between cardiac output and portal venous and hepatic arterial flows. *Hepatol,* 1992;16:715-718

Hoekstra J, Janssen HL. Vascular liver disorders (II): portal vein thrombosis. *Neth J Med,* 2009;67(2):46-53

Janssen HL, Wijnhoud A, Haagsma EB, et al: Extrahepatic portal vein thrombosis: aetiology and determinants of survival. *Gut,* 2001;49:720

Janssen HL. Changing perspectives in portal vein thrombosis. *Scand J Gastroenterol,* 2000;232:69

Jing-Tong W, Hui-Ying Z, Yu-Lan L. Portal vein thrombosis. *Hepatobiliary Pancreat Dis Int,* 2005;4:515-8

Kiladjian JJ, Cervantes F, Leebeek FWG, et al. Role of JAK 2 mutation detection in Budd-Chiari syndrome (BCS) and portal vein thrombosis (PVT) associated to MPD. *Blood,* 2006;108:116a-a

Kocher G, Himmelmann A. Portal vein thrombosis (PVT): a study of 20 non-cirrhotic cases. *Swiss Med Wkly,* 2005;135:372-376

Kutti J, Ridell B. Epidemiology of the myeloproliferative disorders: essential thrombocythemia, polycythaemia vera and idiopathic myelofibrosis. *Pathol Biol,* 2001;49(2):164-6

Landolfi R, Di Gennaro L, Falanga A. Thrombosis in myeloproliferative disorders: pathogenetic facts and speculation. *Leukemia,* 2008;22:2020-2028

Llado L, Fabregat J, Castellote J, et al. Management of portal vein thrombosis in liver transplantation: influence on morbidity and mortality. *Clin Transplant,* 2007;21:716-21

Malkowski P, Pawlak J, Michalowicz B, et al: Thrombolytic treatment of portal thrombosis. *Hepatogastroenterology,* 2003;50:2098

Naonami T, Yokoyama I, Iwatsuki S et al. The incidence of portal vein thrombosis at liver transplantation. *Hepatology,* 1992;169(5):1195-98

Ogren M, Bergqvist D, Bjorck M, et al. Portal vein thrombosis: prevalence, patient characteristics and lifetime risk: a population study based on 23,796 consecutive autopsies. *World J Gastroenterol,* 2006;12:2115-9

Ohnishi K, Okuda K, Ohtsuki T et al. Formation of hilar collateral of or cavernous transformation after portal vein obstruction by hepatocellular carcinoma : observations in ten patients. *Gastroenterol,* 1984;87:1150-53

Perlemuter G, Bejamin H, Fritsch J et al. Biliary obstruction caused by portal cavernoma: a study of 8 cases. *J Hepatol,* 1996;25:58-63

Pirisi M, Avellini C, Fabris C, Scott C, Bardus P, Soardo G, Beltrami CA, Bartoli E. Portal vein thrombosis in hepatocellular carcinoma: age and sex distribution in an autopsy study. *J Cancer Res Clin Oncol,* 1998;124:397-400

Ponziani FR, Zocco MA, Campanale C et al. Portal vein thrombosis: Insight into physiopathology, diagnosis, and treatment. *World J Gastroenterol,* 2010;16(2):143-155

Regev A, Stark P, Blickstein D, et al. Thrombotic complications in essential thrombocythemia with relatively low platelet counts. *Am J Hematol,* 1997;56:168–72

Rollison DE, Howlader N, Smith MT, et al. Epidemiology of myelodysplastic syndromes and chronic myeloproliferative disorders in the United States, 2001-2004, using data from the NAACCR and SEER programs. *Blood,* 2008;112:45-52

Rosendaal FR: Venous thrombosis: a multicausal disease. *Lancet,* 1999;353:1167-1173

Sarin SK, Agarwal SR: Extrahepatic portal vein obstruction. *Semin Liver Dis,* 2002;22:43-58

Sarin SK, Sollano JD, Chawla YK, et al. Consensus on extra-hepatic portal vein obstruction. *Liver Int,* 2006;26:512-519

Sezgin O, Oguz D, Altintas E, Saritas U, Sahin B. Endoscopic management of biliary obstruction caused by cavernous transformation of the portal vein. *Gastrointest Endosc,* 2003;58:602-8

Sobhonslidsuk A, Reddy KR. Portal vein thrombosis: a concise review. *Am J Gastroenterol,* 2002;97:535-541

Søgaard KK, Horváth-Puhó E, Grønbaek H et al. Risk of venous thromboembolism in patients with liver disease: a nationwide population-based case-control study. *Am J Gastroenterol,* 2009;104:96-101

Storen EC, Tefferi A. Long-term use of anagrelide in young patients with essential thrombocythemia. *Blood,* 2001;97:863–6

Tefferi A, Fonseca R, Pereira DL, et al. A long-term retrospective study of young women with essential thrombocythemia. *Mayo Clin Proc,* 2001;76:22–8

Tefferi A, Solberg LA, Silverstein MN. A clinical update in polycythemia vera and essential thrombocythemia. *Am J Med,* 2000;109:141–9

Tefferi A, Thiele J, Orazi A, et al. Proposals and rationale for revision of the World Health Organization diagnostic criteria for polycythemia vera, essential thrombocythemia, and primary myelofibrosis: recommendations from an ad hoc international expert panel. *Blood,* 2007;110:1092–7

Tripodi A, Mannucci PM. The coagulopathy of chronic liver disease. *N Engl J Med,* 2011, 14;365(2):147-56

Ueno N, Sasaki A, Tomiyama T, et al. Color Doppler ultrasonography in the diagnosis of cavernous transformation of the portal vein. *J Clin Ultrasound,* 1997;25:227-33

Valla DC, Casadevall N, Huisse MG, Tulliez M. Etiology of portal vein thrombosis in adults. A prospective evaluation of primary myeloproliferative disorders. *Gastroenterology,* 1988;94:1063-9

Valla DC, Condat B. Portal vein thrombosis in adults: pathophysiology, pathogenesis and management. *J Hepatol,* 2000;32:865-71

Valla DC, Condat B, Lebrec D. Spectrum of portal vein thrombosis in the West. *J Gastroenterol Hepatol,* 2002;17:s224

Vibert E, Azoulay D, Castaing D, Bismuth H. Portal cavernoma: diagnosis, aetiologies and consequences. *Ann Chir,* 2002;127:745-750

Walker AP: Portal vein thrombosis: what is the role of genetics? *Eur J Gastroenterol Hepatol,* 2005;17:705-707

Wang JT, Zhao HY, Liu YL. Portal vein thrombosis. *Hepatobiliary Pancreat Dis Int,* 2005;4:515-518

Webster GJ, Burroughs AK, Riordan SM: Review article: portal vein thrombosis - new insights into aetiology and management. *Aliment Pharmacol Ther,* 2005;21:1-9

5

The Bacterial Endotoxins Levels in the Blood of Cirrhotic Patients as Predictor of the Risk of Esophageal Varices Bleeding

Dmitry Garbuzenko, Alexandr Mikurov
and Dmitry Smirnov
*Department of Surgical Diseases and Urology,
Chelyabinsk State Medical Academy,
Russia*

1. Introduction

In cirrhotic patients the bleeding from esophageal varices is the most dangerous complication of portal hypertension and is attended with high rate of lethality. Endoscopic assessment of esophageal varices and the state of esophageal and stomach mucosa at the esophagogastroduodenoscopy presents high importance for the assessment of risk of their development (Coelho-Prabhu & Kamath, 2010). However, invasiveness as well as discomfort that are tolerated by patients during the given procedure, lead to the rejection from it and therefore they can't be subjected to examination in a number of cases. Besides, the research might be impossible to carry out in case if the state of patient is grave (de Franchis et al., 2008). The investigation of hepatic venous pressure gradient, that reflects the portal hypertension intensity best of all haven`t been realized in the clinical practice up to now (Groszmann et al., 2006). Considering the above mentioned disadvantages of main methods, the development of additional prognostic criteria of the risk of esophageal varices bleeding remains the urgent problem of the internal medicine (Cárdenas & Ginès, 2009).

Over the last years the greatest importance in the development of the given complication is placed to the endotoxemia as a result of the translocation of gram-negative bacteria from intestinal tube (Boursier et al., 2007). It was demonstrated that the latter presents the important part of the hyperdynamic circulatory status at the portal hypertension and also lies in the basis of hepatocellular insufficiency and brings about the haemostasis disorder in cirrhotic patients (Thalheimer et al., 2005). Besides, it was reported that bacteremia often accompanies esophageal varices bleeding (Lata et al., 2005), decreases the efficiency of the conservative or endoscopic therapy (Zhao et al., 2002) and bears the risk factor for recurrent bleeding (Brown et al., 2010).

The aim of the research is to illustrate the appropriateness of the assessment of the bacterial endotoxins levels in the blood of cirrhotic patients as the method to predict the risk of esophageal varices bleeding.

2. Patients and methods

The prospective incidence research has been carried out that covers 90 cirrhotic patients with portal hypertension between September 2008 and December 2010 at our clinic (The department of surgical diseases and urology, Chelyabinsk State Medical Academy, Chelyabinsk, Russia). Only patients with esophageal varices was included in the study. All patients underwent a detailed clinical evaluation, including blood tests, ultrasonography, esophagogastroduodenoscopy. Moreover the quality and quantity assessment of endotoxemia intensity was performed.

2.1 Blood tests

Hematological and biochemical work-up included measurement of hemoglobin, total leukocyte count, platelet count, serum concentrations of bilirubin (total and conjugated), protein, albumin, alanine aminotransferase and aspartate aminotrasferase. Furthermore the hemostatic factors of their peripheral blood, such as prothrombin time, International Normalized Ratio, activated partial thromboplastin time, activated recalcification time, soluble fibrin-monomer complexes, fibrinogen, Hageman factor dependent fibrinolysis, were examined. For each patient, a modified Child-Pugh score was calculated (Pugh et al., 1973). All patients were tested for HBV-DNA, HBeAg, HBsAg, anti-HBcAg, antibodies to hepatitis C virus, antimitochondrial antibodies to determine the cause of liver cirrhosis.

2.2 Ultrasound Doppler

All patients underwent ultrasonography and the follow details were recorded: Maximum vertical span of the liver, nodularity of liver surface; spleen size (length of its longest axis); diametr of the portal and splenic veins; presence of portal-systemic collaterals; and presence of ascites.

The portal vein was imaged longitudinally in the supine position, and the Doppler sample volume was set at the midpoint between the confluence of the splenic and superior mesenteric vein and the bifurcation of the portal vein at the hepatic hilus. When the sample point was adjusted to the center of the portal vein, the portal venous velocity was recorded in a quiet suspended expiration and was averaged over a few seconds. Portal venous flow was determined by the formula, cross-sectional area × mean velocity × 60 (Choi et al., 2003). The mean velocity of the splenic vein was determined using the same method as used for the portal vein.

2.3 Endoscopic evaluation

All patients underwent esophagogastroduodenoscopy for assessment of esophageal varices, the degree of which was defined according to the international classification offered by Japanese Research Society for Portal Hypertension (Japanese Research Society for Portal Hypertension, 1980): F0 – absent; F1 – straight; F2 – winding; F3 – nodule-beaded.

2.4 Assessment of endotoxemia intensity

To make the quality and quantity assessment of endotoxemia intensity their blood was collected into a sterile test tube without anticoagulants, it was placed into the thermostat for

30-40 minutes with the temperature of 37° C and then centrifugated during 15 minutes at 3000 revolution per minute. The obtained serosity was used for analysis during 2 hours. In a number of case it was possible to apply cold singly and store it.

Abacterial express-diagnostics of common endotoxin of gram-negative bacteria was conducted by the method of activated particles (MAP) with the test sets "MAP - Endotox spp.", developed in Research center of cardiovascular surgery named after A.N. Bakulev, Russian Academy of Medical Sciences and Research and Production Company "Rokhat" (Bokeriia et al., 2007). The given method is based on immobilization of polymer chemical microspheres with a size of particle equal to 0,62 - 0,68 micron of monoclonal antibodies, subclass IqG 3 and IqG 2a, 0:111 B4 J5. The reaction accounting was maintained considering the degree of particle activation (DPA) in the diagnostic titer 1:8 on point-based system ranging from 1 to 4.

The levels of endotoxemia is determined by means of turbidimetric test on the end point that serves as a variant of Limulus lysate amebocyte assay (LAL-assay), firstly described in 1968 by J. Levin and F.B. Bang (Levin J. & Bang F.B., 1968). Its basis is formed by the ability of Lymulus amebocyte lysate react with endotoxins (liposaccharides) of gram-negative bacteria in a specific way. The amount of bacterial endotoxin contained in the examined samples was determined according the pharmacopoeial techniques that were attached to the set of chemical reagents produced by the "LAL Center" (Moscow, Russia). The analysis was carried out on microtitration plates with the application of photoelectric colorimeter "Multi Scan". The measurement were made at the length of wave equal to 405 millimicron. Calibration curve was built using three-four known concentrations of control standard endotoxin.

2.5 Statistical analysis

The statistical analysis of the data received was conducted with the help of program package "Statistica 5.5". We calculated values M, their standard mistakes (m) and 95 % of confidence interval, and used non-parametric Mann and Whitney test. Besides, we applied Spirmen coefficient of rank correlation. The differences were considered to be accurate at $P < 0,05$.

3. Results

Ninety cirrhotic patients with portal hypertension were enrolled in this study, with a median age of 46,2 ± 20 years. There were 47 men and 43 women. Both the virus and alcohol were the aetiology of liver cirrhosis in 18 patients. Primary biliary cirrhosis was found in 3 patients. It was not possible to establish the cause of disease in 51 cases. Hepatocellular insufficiency according to Child-Pugh score was grade A in 18 patients, grade B in 52 patients, grade C in 20 patients.

Esophagogastroduodenoscopy demonstrated esophageal varices of first degree (F1) in 17 patients, of second degree (F2) in 52 patients, of third degree (F3) in 21 patients. Sixty-five had gastro-esophageal bleeding due to variceal rupture. Patients were divided into 3 groups: first group (25 people) was presented by the patients without esophageal varices bleeding, the second group (20 people) consisted of those who had tolerated it in the medical background, the third group (45 people) - was made by patients in the urgent order with esophageal varices bleeding.

In the framework of both the quality and quantity assessment of endotoxemia there were the statistically significant differences obtained between the groups put in contrast (P < 0,05). Thus, its intensity, determined by the method of particles activation turned out to be the most significant for the patients with esophageal varices bleeding, and appeared to be the minimal with people not suffering from such a complication (Table 1).

Groups of patients		Endotoxemia levels			
		1 DPA	2 DPA	3 DPA	4 DPA
I	Without esophageal varices bleeding	N = 20	N = 5	0	0
II	Esophageal varices bleeding in the medical history	N = 5	N = 10	N = 5	0
III	Acute esophageal varices bleeding	0	N = 5	N = 11	N = 29

Notice. Spirmen coefficient (R = 0,82; P < 0,05; N = 90).

DPA - degree of particle activation.

Table 1. Qualitative assessment of the endotoxemia intensity in cirrhotic patients with portal hypertension (MAP – Endotox test; DPA)

The levels of bacterial endotoxins in the blood of patients that had arrived in the order of emergency varied between 4,1 to 59,1 ng/ml and was authentically higher (p<0,05) than of patients without or with the variceal bleeding in the medical background: from 0 to 0,8 ng/ml and from 1,3 to 2,3 ng/ml, respectively (Table 2).

Groups of patients		
Without esophageal varices bleeding	Esophageal varices bleeding in the medical history	Acute esophageal varices bleeding
I	II	III
0,5 ± 0,1 N = 25	1,9 ± 0,1 N = 25 P(I – II)*	32,1 ± 3,0 N = 45 P(I - III)* P(II - III)*

Notice: P()* - difference between contrast groups are statistically significant.
U-criterion of Mann and Whitney applied; P < 0,05.
LAL-assay - Limulus lysate amebocyte assay.

Table 2. The bacterial endotoxins levels in the blood of cirrhotic patients with portal hypertension (ng/ml) (LAL-assay), M ± m

With 13 patients without the previous record of variceal bleeding, the latter appeared in a period of 3-4 days later from the moment of planned hospitalization. In all cases there was the increased levels of bacterial endotoxins in the blood recorded as early as the very moment of admittance to hospital (8,3 ± 3,9 ng/ml), at the time of bleeding it increased to 38,7 ± 4,6 ng/ml (p<0,05), and 5-7 days later after achieving the effective hemostasis it decreased to 3,2 ± 1,6 ng/ml (P < 0,05).

Among the patients admitted with acute esophageal varices bleeding, 16 of them had its early recurrence in the upcoming 24 hours after the primary hemostasia. They all had a high levels of bacterial endotoxins in blood (36,2 ± 6,7 ng/ml) which having decreased down to 6,8 ± 2,5 ng/ml (P < 0,05) against the background of conservative therapy, sharply rose to 39,3 ± 6,3 ng/ml at the blooding recurrence. When the stable hemostasis had been achieved its values decreased down to 3,1 ± 1,1 ng/ml (P < 0,05).

Presuming that the minimal concentration of bacterial endotoxins in the blood of those who suffer from the acute esophageal varices bleeding made 4,1 ng/ml and the maximal value among those who were admitted to hospital routinely comprised 2,3 ng/ml, we had the opportunity to determine the intervals of values endotoxemia according to the degree of esophageal varices bleeding risk. Considering the fact that the levels of bacterial endotoxins in the blood of the selected patients (90 people) ranging from 0 to 4,0 ng/ml determed the low possibility of complication occurrence and the values above 4,1 ng/ml confirmed the high risk, the diagnostic criterion 4,0 ng/ml turned out to be the best one. The sensitivity and specificity was 90 % and 85 % respectively.

From 45 patients that were admitted to hospitals with acute bleeding, only 2 patients had the esophageal varices of the first degree whereas 23 and 20 patients were found to suffer from the esophageal varices of the second and third degree correspondingly. On the opposite, among 45 patients that were hospitalized routinely the esophageal varices of the first degree was identified in 15 cases; of the second degree - found in 26 patients, and as for the third - only with 4 of them.

At the quality assessment of endotoxemia in case of all the patients involved in research, there is the credible correlation (P < 0,05) between its parameters, the degree of esophageal varices and the bleeding occurrence. Thus, if in case of patients with acute bleeding with esophageal varices mainly of 2-3 degrees (43 people), the intensity of endotoxemia seemed significant, its intensity was insignificant among the patients with esophageal varices of 1-2 degrees (41 people) as a rule, admitted without such complication (Table 3).

Esophageal varices			Endotoxemia levels			
			1 DPA	2 DPA	3 DPA	4 DPA
Acute esophageal varices bleeding	No	F1	10	4	1	0
		F2	15	10	1	0
		F3	0	1	3	0
	Yes	F1	0	1	1	0
		F2	0	4	10	9
		F3	0	0	0	20

Notice. Spirmen coefficient (R = 0,87; P < 0,05; N = 90).
MAP - method of activated particles.
DPA - degree of particle activation.

Table 3. The correlation between the intensity of endotoxemia in cirrhotic patients, the degree of esophageal varices and the availability of acute bleeding from them (MAP – Endotox test; DPA)

In order to carry out the correlation analysis of bacterial endotoxins levels in the blood, the degree of esophageal varices and the acute bleeding occurrence the patients were divided into four subgroups. The patients with esophageal varices of the first degree without acute bleeding made subgroup A. Since the intensity of endotoxemia in the patients with esophageal varices of the second and the third degree, admitted without the mentioned complication was similar and a number of the latter minor we combined into one subgroup B. For this very reason the patients were combined suffering from esophageal varices of the first and second degree, hospitalized with acute bleeding (subgroup C). Those who were admitted in the emergency order with the same diagnosis as well as the esophageal varices of the third degree made subgroup D.

The data received corresponded to the quality values and were statistically accurate (P < 0,05). There was also the direct correlation dependence observed between the levels of bacterial endotoxins in the blood, the degree of esophageal varices and the availability of acute bleeding from them. Thus, the endotoxemia was least pronounced in the patients of subgroup A: ranging from 0 to 0,8 ng/ml and mostly identified in subgroup D: from 29,4 to 59,1 ng/ml. In subgroups B and C: from 0,9 to 2,3 ng/ml and from 9,8 to 19,9 ng/ml, correspondingly (Table 4).

Groups of patients			
Without acute esophageal varices bleeding		With acute esophageal varices bleeding	
Subgroup A	Subgroup B	Subgroup C	Subgroup D
0,03 ± 0,01 N = 15	1,2 ± 0,8 N = 30 P(A-B)*	14,9 ± 5,0 N = 25 P(A-C)*; P(B-C)*	34,3 ± 4,7 N = 20 P(A-D)*; P(B-D)*; P(C-D)*

Notice: P()* - difference between the contrast subgroups are statistically significant. U-criterion of Mann and Whitney applied; P < 0,05.
LAL-assay - Limulus lysate amebocyte assay.

Table 4. The correlation between the bacterial endotoxins levels in the blood of cirrhotic patients, the degree of esophageal varices and the availability of acute bleeding from them (ng/ml) (LAL-assay), M ± m

4. Discussion

In cirrhotic patients the bleeding from esophageal varices is a serious and potentially life-threatening complication of portal hypertension. The risk of bleeding can be reduced nearly by half by appropriate prophylactic therapy (de Franchis, R. & Baveno V Faculty, 2010), which has prompted the identification of noninvasive indicators of esophageal varices, aimed to decrease the need for screening endoscopy, which is currently recommended in all cirrhotic patients at the time of diagnosis. Low platelet count, splenomegaly, a portal vein diametr on ultrasound ≥ 13 mm, a high Child-Pugh score, low ptothrombin activity, the presence of spider angiomas, and a low platelet to spleen ratio have been the parameters most frequently associated with presence varices and the risk of bleeding from them (Berzigotti A. et al., 2008). Endotoxaemia is frequently found in cirrhotic patients, even in the absence of any signs of sepsis. Thus higher endotoxins concentrations are found in peripheral blood of cirrhotics than in normal subjects with a statistically significant gradient between portal and peripheral blood, highlighting the role of the bowel as the source of endotoxins. Both peripheral and portal levels of endotoxaemia are correlated with the severity of liver disease which is a more important predictor of high plasma endotoxins concentrations than portosystemic shunting or portal hypertension (Lin R.S. et al., 1995). Further, plasma levels of the bacterial endotoxins in cirrhotic patients were significantly positively associated with hepatic venous pressure gradient, wedge hepatic venous pressure, and hepatic sinusoid resistance (Lee K.C., 2010).

We evaluated of the bacterial endotoxins levels in the blood of cirrhotic patients as the method to predict the risk of esophageal varices bleeding. Our study detected that the highest manifestation of endotoxemia in cirrhotic patients is observed in case of acute bleeding from the esophageal varices. With the patients that had bleeding in the medical background, its values exceed the values of those who hadn`t this complication.

While the bacterial endotoxins levels in the blood of cirrhotic patients ranging from 0 to 4,0 ng/ml determines the low possibility of bleeding occurrence, the values exceeding 4,1 ng/ml demonstrate its high risk probability. Accordingly, diagnostics criterion of 4,0 ng/ml appears to be the most adequate and relevant one. The sensitivity and specificity was 90 % and 85 % respectively.

Moreover we found that the intensity of endotoxemia with cirrhotic patients adequately correlate with the degree of esophageal varices and the bleeding occurrence in them.

5. Conclusion

Notwithstanding the fact that the main predictor of the risk of esophageal varices bleeding in cirrhotic patients is endoscopic assessment of their intensity according to data of esophagogastroduodenoscopy, in case if its fulfillment appears to be impossible (if a patient rejects the research being made, if the condition of a patient is grave and so on) the detection of the bacterial endotoxins serum levels can serve as the alternative prognostic index. Further validation of the results will be achieved through long-term follow-up of the patients and a larger number of studied subjects.

6. References

Berzigotti, A.; Gilabert, R.; Abraldes, J.G.; Nicolau, C.; Bru, C.; Bosch, J. & García-Pagan, J.C. Noninvasive prediction of clinically significant portal hypertension and esophageal varices in patients with compensated liver cirrhosis. *Am J Gastroenterol,* Vol.103, №8, (August 2008), pp. 1159-1167

Bokeriia, L.A.; Serov, V.N.; Sarkisov, S.E.; Karamishev, V.K.; Volovikov, L.V. & Niyazmatov, A.A. (2007). Express-diagnostics of endotoxin of gram-negative bacteria in gynecologic practic. *Akush Ginekol (Moskow),* №1, (January 2007), pp. 28-30

Boursier, J.; Asfar, P.; Joly-Guillou, M.L. & Cales., P. (2007). Infection and variceal bleeding in cirrhosis. *Gastroenterol Clin Biol,* Vol.31, №1, (January 2007), pp. 27-38

Brown, M.R.; Jones, G.; Nash, K.L.; Wright, M. & Guha, I.N. (2010). Antibiotic prophylaxis in variceal hemorrhage: timing, effectiveness and Clostridium difficile rates. *World J Gastroenterol,* Vol.16, №42, (November 2010), pp. 5317-5323

Cárdenas, A. & Ginès, P. (2009). Portal hypertension. *Curr Opin Gastroenterol,* Vol.25, №3, (May 2009), pp. 195-201

Choi, Y.J.; Baik, S.K.; Park, D.H.; Kim, M.Y.; Kim, H.S.; Lee, D.K.; Kwon, S.O.; Kim, Y.J. & Park, J.W. (2003). Comparison of Doppler ultrasonography and the hepatic venous pressure gradient in assessing portal hypertension in liver cirrhosis. *J Gastroenterol Hepatol,* Vol.18, №4, (April 2003), pp. 424-429

Coelho-Prabhu, N. & Kamath, P.S. (2010). Current staging and diagnosis of gastroesophageal varices. *Clin Liver Dis,* Vol.14, №2, (May 2010), pp. 195-208

de Franchis, R.; Eisen, G.M.; Laine, L.; Fernandez-Urien, I.; Herrerias, J.M.; Brown, R.D.; Fisher, L.; Vargas, H.E.; Vargo, J.; Thompson, J. & Eliakim, R. (2008). Esophageal capsule endoscopy for screening and surveillance of esophageal varices in patients with portal hypertension. *Hepatology,* Vol.47, №5, (May 2008), pp. 1595-1603

de Franchis, R. & Baveno V Faculty (2010). Revising consensus in portal hypertension: report of the Baveno V consensus workshop on methodology of diagnosis and therapy in portal hypertension. *J Hepatol,* Vol.53, №4, (October 2010), pp. 762-768

Groszmann, R.; Vorobioff, J.D. & Gao, H. (2006). Measurement of portal pressure: when, how, and why to do it. *Clin Liver Dis,* Vol.10, №3, (August 2006), pp. 499-512

Japanese Research Society for Portal Hypertension (1980). The general rules for recording endoscopic findings on esophageal varices. *Jpn J Surg,* Vol.10, №1, (March 1980), pp. 84-87

Lata, J.; Juránková, J.; Husová, L.; Senkyrík, M.; Díte, P.; Dastych, M.; Príbramská, V. & Kroupa, R. (2005). Variceal bleeding in portal hypertension: bacterial infection and comparison of efficacy of intravenous and per-oral application of antibiotics - a randomized trial. *Eur J Gastroenterol Hepatol,* Vol.17, №10, (October 2005), pp. 1105-1110

Lee, K.C.; Yang, Y.Y.; Wang, Y.W.; Lee, F.A.; Loong, C.C.; Hou, M.C.; Lin, H.C. & Lee, S.D. (2010). Increased plasma malondialdehyde in patients with viral cirrhosis and its relationships to plasma nitric oxide, endotoxin, and portal pressure. *Dig Dis Sci,* Vol.55, №7, (July 2010), pp. 2077-2085

Levin, J. & Bang, F.B. (1968). Clottable protein in Limulus; its localization and kinetics of its coagulation by endotoxin. *Thromb Diath Haemorrh,* Vol.19, №1, (March 1968), pp. 186-197

Lin, R.S.; Lee, F.Y.; Lee, S.D.; Tsai, Y.T.; Lin, H.C.; Lu, R.H.; Hsu, W.C.; Huang, C.C.; Wang, S.S. & Lo, K.J. (1995). Endotoxemia in patients with chronic liver diseases: relationship to severity of liver diseases, presence of esophageal varices, and hyperdynamic circulation. *J Hepatol,* Vol.22, №2, (February 1995), pp. 165-172

Pugh, R.N.H.; Murray-Lyon, I.M.; Dawson, J.R.; Pietroni, M.C. & Williams, R. (1973). Transection of the oesophagus for bleeding oesophageal varices. *Br J Surg,* Vol.60, №8, (August 1973), pp. 646-649

Thalheimer, U.; Triantos, C.K.; Samonakis, D.N.; Patch, D. & Burroughs, A.K. (2005). Infection, coagulation, and variceal bleeding in cirrhosis. *Gut,* Vol.54, №4, (April 2005), pp. 556-563

Zhao, C.; Chen, S.B.; Zhou, J.P.; Xiao, W.; Fan, H.G.; Wu, X.W.; Feng, G.X. & He, W.X. (2002). Prognosis of hepatic cirrhosis patients with esophageal or gastric variceal hemorrhage: multivariate analysis. *Hepatobiliary Pancreat Dis Int,* Vol.1, №3, (August 2002), pp. 416-419

6

Traditional Chinese Medicine Can Improve Liver Microcirculation and Reduce Portal Hypertension in Liver Cirrhosis

Xu Lieming[1,5], Gu Jie[2], Lu Xiong[2], Zhou Yang[1,5], Tian Tian[2], Zhang Jie[2] and Xu Hong[2]
[1]*Shuguang Hospital Affiliated to Shanghai University of Traditional Chinese Medicine,*
[2]*Institute of Liver Diseases, Shanghai University of TCM*
[3]*Key Laboratory of Liver and Kidney Diseases, Ministry of Education*
[4]*Key Laboratory of Traditional Chinese Medicine Clinic, Shanghai*
[5]*The Key Unit of Liver Diseases, SATCM. Shanghai, China*

1. Introduction

Liver microcirculation means that the blood circulation is sinusoids as a center, from the end branch of portal vein and hepatic artery through sinusoids to central vein in the liver. Liver microcirculation has two characteristics. One character is there are two import systems from portal vein and hepatic artery. Another is sinusoids with unique structure. All blood vessels which diameters are less 300μm are part of microcirculation system. These vessels are able to regulate the blood flow and distribution.[1]

Sinusoids are a capillary bed which is major place for regulation of blood and exchange of material in the liver. Sinusoids are constituted by microvasculature, sinusoid endothelial cells (SEC), Kupffer cells (KC) and hepatic stellate cells (HSC). [2] SEC and HSC are considered as cellular factors for regulation of sinusoids blood flow. HSC is located in perisinusoids with functions include storing Vitamin A, and controlling the diameter and blood flow of sinusoids by its pseudopods around sinusoids.[3] SEC, KC and HSC all have contractility because they contain fiber, microvasculature and contractile protein.[2]

The liver complex functions, which are biological synthesis, metabolism, detoxify and host defense, are tightly dependent perfect liver microcirculation.[4] It is showed that failure of liver microcirculation is a general pathological alteration in chronic hepatitis and liver cirrhosis because changed construction of microvasculature, capillarization of sinusoid (the collagen is filled in perisinusoids) and compression of fibrous tissue. Generally, stenosis of sinusoid will lead to increase of resistence, decrease of blood flow rate and flow volume, and formation of portal hypertension. It is indicated that after hepatitis B virus infection, platelets were recruited to the liver, and their activation correlated with severely reduced sinusoidal microcirculation, delayed virus elimination and increased immunopathological liver cell damage.[5]

In normal condition, liver microcirculation is regulated by 3 ways. (1) SEC is a regulator of blood flow in the liver. The liver injury will lead to injury of SEC, reduction of fenestrae in SEC, straitens of sinusoid within accumulation of erythrocytes and formation of microthrombus. Injury and necrosis of SEC are major causes of disorder of liver microcirculation. (2) KC can also regulate the liver blood flow by its pseudopod inner of sinusoid. Actived KC may lead stenosis of sinusoid due to conglutination of leukocytes.[6] (3) HSC is able to directly regulate contraction of sinusoids in normal liver. Active HSC has stronger character of contraction with increased concentration of Ca^{2+}. HSC is just located in the site of sinusoid contraction. Propotional relationship has been proved between contraction of HSC and activation of HSC both *in vivo* and *in vitro*.[7,8] Many chemical compounds are as inductors to induce contraction of HSC. They are included Endothelin-1 (ET-1), Angiotensin II and vasopressin. ET-1 is concerned a strongest cytokine to induce contraction of HSC. Perfusion of ET-1 through portal vein leads to contraction of sinusoids. However, the compounds of NO, CO and adrenal medullar hormone have the functions to against ET-1-stimulated contraction of HSC. Contraction of active HSC (myofibroblast cell), which locates in fibrous septum in cirrhotic liver, can change construction of hepatic lobule and lead to increase resistens of microcirculation in the liver.

Once failure of microcirculation in the liver, some symptoms and signs of patient are similar "blood stasis" in Traditional Chinese Medicine. Those are twinge in inside right flank or rib, hepatomegaly or splenomegaly, dim complexion, accompanied with spider nevi and liver palms, deep-red tongue, ecchymosis, taut or thready pulse. Some Chinese herb medicine, which is able to promote blood circulation to remove blood stasis, can prevent esophageal variceal bleeding on cirrhotic patients with portal hypertension, improve liver microcirculation and decrease portal hypertension through treating cirrhotic rats *in vivo* and inhibit contraction of active HSC *in vitro* in resent 10 years.[9]

Fuzheng Huayu Capsule (FZHYC), a traditional Chinese medicine recipe, has demonstrated the effect of anti-fibrosis and reduced portal vein pressure in patients with chronic hepatitis B.[10] Fuzheng means supporting the healthy energy. Huayu means dispersing blood stasis. The recipe is composed by 6 herbs those are Dan Shen (*Radix Salviae Miltiorrhizae*), Chong Cao (*Paecilomyces hepiali Chen & Dai*), Tao Ren (*Semen Persicae*), Jiao Gu Lan (*Gynostemma pentaphyllum*), Song Hua Fen (*Pinus armandii Franch*) and Wu Wei Zi (*Fructus Schisandrae Chinensis*). FZHYC has been used in numerous studies in China and has been found to have a satisfactory prophylaxis effect on the chronic liver injury and hepatic fibrosis in rats and humans. In addition, it enhances hepatic fibrolysis.[11]

2. The clinical research

2.1 Aims

To elucidate the role of FZHYC in the prevention of esophageal variceal bleeding on cirrhotic patients with portal hypertension.

2.2 Methods

In a multi-center randomized and placebo-controlled trial, 146 cirrhotic patients, whose age range was between 18 and 70 years old, with esophageal varices were enrolled. According to the degree of esophageal and gastric varices, patients were stratified as 2 levels: small level, and moderate and severe level. The randomization code was generated by SAS software for each subject. For patients with small varices, the trial was double blinded. The patients were randomly assigned to 2 groups: Patients were treated with FZHYC in FZHYC group or received placebo in control group. For patients with moderate and severe varices, the trial was single blind. They were divided into 3 groups: FZHYC group in which patients were treated with FZHYC, propranolol group in which patients were treated with Propranolol and combination group in which patients received both FZHYC and propranolol. The dose of FZHYC was 15 capsules (0.3g per capsule) per day and orally administrated at 3 times. The placebo was composed of stir-fried wheat powder with an identical-appearance in the aspects of dosage, color of the contents and packaging. The clinical intervention period lasts 2 years and the follow up would stop once the end points occur. The primary end point was esophageal or gastric variceal bleeding.

2.3 Results

2.3.1 In patients with small varices level

A total of 6 patients reached the primary end point of esophageal variceal bleeding: 1 of 29 patients in the Fuzheng Huayu group and 5 of 27 patients in the control group. The actuarial probability of remaining free of esophageal variceal bleeding was a significant different between 2 groups (96.3% vs. 77.01%, P=0.0422) (Fig. 1). Some patients with small varices were willing to be re-examined by endoscopy after treatment and small varices was dispared in several patients. There was a significant difference of esophageal varices degree in FZHYC group compared to the control group (P=0.014). (Tab. 1 and Fig. 2).

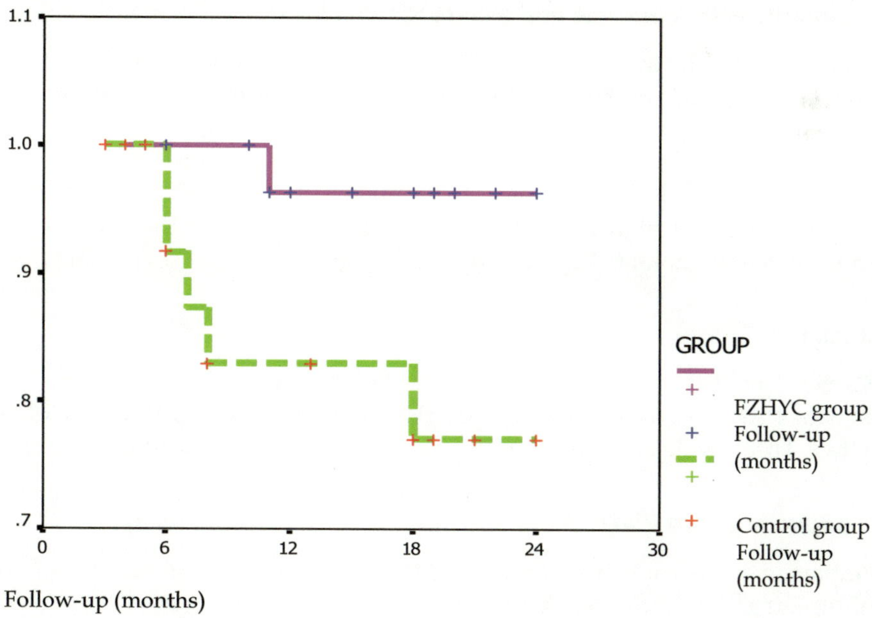

Fig. 1. Actuarial probability of remaining free of esophageal variceal bleeding in cirrhotic patients with small varices level. The patients were treated with Fuzheng Huayu Capsule in FZHYC group or placebo in control group for 24 months. Actuarial probability of remaining free of esophageal variceal bleeding was higher in FZHYC group than in controls (P<0.05).

Groups	n	No varices (n)	No changes (n)	Enlarged varices (n)
FZHYC *	15	8	5	2
control	9	1	3	5

Note: compared with control group,*: P=0.014

Table 1. Difference of developing small varices in FZHYC group and in controls after 24 months

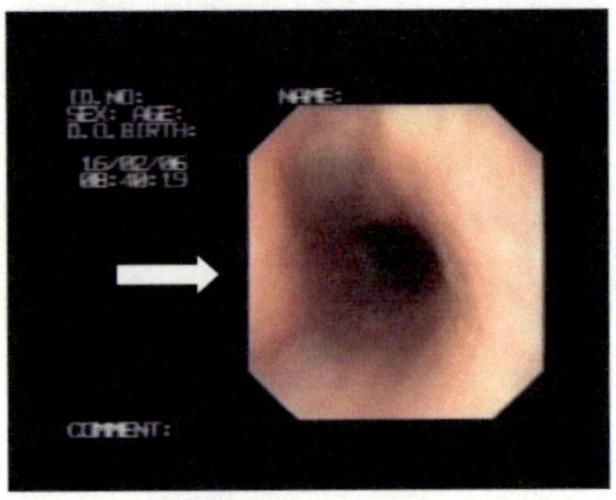

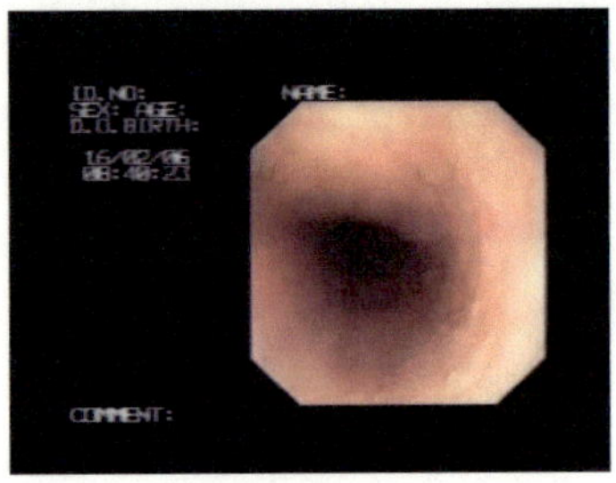

pre treatment **post treatment**

Fig. 2. Alteration of small varices by endoscopy examination at pre and post treatment of FZHYC. Arrow shows the small varices in a cirrhotic patient at pre treatmtnt (left). The small varices, however, was disappeared in same patient at post treatmtnt (right).

2.3.2 In patients with moderate and severe varices level

5 patients in FZHYC group (n=30), 8 patients in Propranolol group (n=30) and 3 patients in the combination group (n=30) had esophageal variceal bleeding during their follow-up. Compared to the Propranolol group (56.99%), there were significant differences in the actuarial probability of remaining free of esophageal variceal bleeding in FZHYC group (76.13%, P=0.0131) and the combination group (87.55%, P=0.0086). Remaining free of variceal bleeding has a higher trend in combination group, but there was no significant difference between combination group and FZHYC group (P=0.3876) (Fig.3).

2.4 Summary

FZHYC could effectively reduce the risk of esophageal variceal bleeding for cirrhotic patients with varices; especially the combination of the capsule and Propranolol delivered a better effect. The capsule could reduce the varices size in patients with small ones.

3. The experiment *in vivo*

For studying the mechanism of Fuzheng Huayu Capsule on prevention of esophageal variceal bleeding, we performed several experiments. *Radix Salviae Miltiorrhizae* is a major herb medicine in Fuzheng Huayu Recipe. Salvianolic-acid B (SA-B), which was extracted from *Radix Salviae Miltiorrhizae,* has been demonstrated to inhibit proliferation and functions of HSC *in vitro* [12]and anti-fibrosis *in vivo.*[13] We did lot of work to deal with how Fuzheng Huayu Recipe and SA-B relieves portal hypertension.

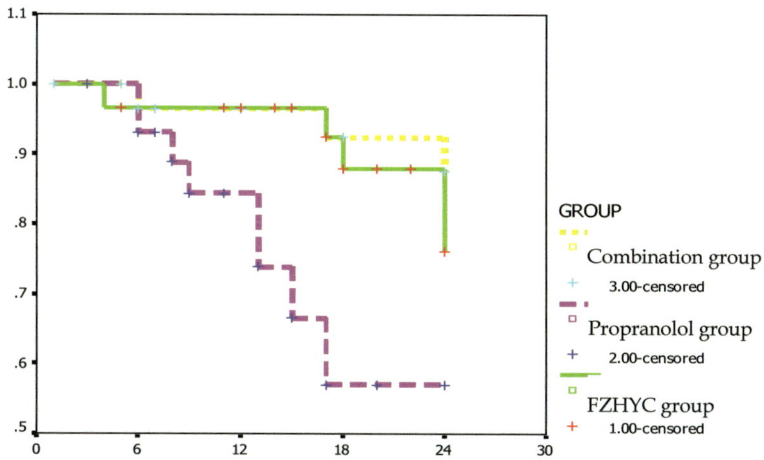

Fig. 3. Actuarial probability of remaining free of esophageal variceal bleeding in cirrhotic patients with moderate and severe varices level The patients were treated with Fuzheng Huayu Capsule in FZHYC group, Propranolol in Propranolol group, or hoth in combination group for 24 months. Actuarial probability of remaining free of esophageal variceal bleeding was higher in combination group and FZHYC group than in Propranolol group. Compared with Propranolol group, the difference was significant in combination group (P<0.01) and in FZHYC group (P<0.05). Although the probability was higher in combination group than in FZHYC group, but the difference was not significant.

3.1 Experiment 1: Chinese herb medicine can decrease portal vein pressure in cirrhotic rats

3.1.1 Aims

To investigate effect of Fuzheng Huayu Recipe and SA-B on decreasing portal vein pressure in cirrhotic rats.

3.1.2 Methods

3.1.2.1 Establishment of liver cirrhosis model

The Sprague-Dawley male rats were randomly divided into model group (n=46) and normal group (n=14).The rats in model group were administrated intraperitoneally with 0.5% dimethylnitrosamine (DMN) at a dose of 2ml/kg body weight for 3 consecutive days and interval 4 days per week. The treatment was for 4 weeks. The rats in normal group were administrated intraperitoneally with physiological salin at a dose of 2ml/kg body weight for same duration.

3.1.2.2 Grouping animals and drug administration

After molding, two rats were randomly sacrificed to observe pathological changes of the liver tissue. The rats in model group were randomly more divided into 3 groups, control group (n=13), Fuzheng Huayu (FZHY) group (n=15) and the SA-B group (n=16), once liver cirrhosis was confirmed. The rats in the FZHY group were gavaged with extractor of Fuzheng Huayu Recipe. The content of extractor equals 36.9g crude drug per 100ml. The rats in the SA-B group were gavaged with SA-B solution (125mg per 100ml). Simultaneously, the rats in control group and normal group were gavaged with water. All dose of gavage was 1ml/100g body weight, once per day, for 3 weeks.

3.1.2.3 Measurement of portal vein pressure

The rats were anesthetized with 2% sodium pentobarbital (2ml/kg body weight) in the end of experiment. One PE-10 tube filling with heparin was inserted from superior mesenteric vein into portal vein and then connected with pressotransducer to measure pressure. Enterocoelia was exposed totally after mesurement. If ascites was found, dry cotton ball was used to blot liquid and then it was weighted for measurement of ascites. Serum separated from blood which was taken in the vena cava was used for liver function detection. The sample of liver tissue, which was 1.0cm×0.8cm×0.3cm, was fixed by formalin, embedded by paraffin, and cutted for 4μm thick for HE and collagen staining. Moreover, 100mg liver tissue was used to detect hydroxyproline (Hyp).

3.1.3 Result

3.1.3.1 Investigating death and ascites in the rats

During making hepatic cirrhosis model, there were no dead rats in week 4 but the death started in week 5. Until the end of week 7, there was still no death in normal group but there were 4 dead rats in control group, 2 dead rats both in FZHY group and in SA-B group, respectively. The reason that leads to death was liver failure. The number of the rats with ascites was most in control group than in other groups. The difference was significantly. (Tab. 2)

Groups	n	Death（n）	Ascites（n）
normal	14	0	0
control	13	4	6
FZHY	15	2	1*
SA-B	16	2	0*

Note: compared with control group, *: $P<0.05$

Table 2. The situation of death and ascites in cirrhotic rats in each group

3.1.3.2 Observation of Pathology of liver in rats

3.1.3.2.1 Inflammation was reduced by Chinese herb medicine in the liver of cirrhotic rats

The structure of liver lobule was clear, hepatocytes arranged as cords radially from central vein to the periphery and a few connective tissue was observed in the portal area in normal group. At the end of treatment, pathological alteration was observed in the liver that was large bleeding area, a lot of swell or necrotic hepatocytes, a lot of infiltrating inflammatory cells including lymphocytes and mononuclears, distorted sinusoids and obviously widened portal areas in controls. They were varying decreased that was degeneration or necrosis of hepatocytes, and intrahepatic hemorrhage both in FZHY group and in SA-B group compared with controls. (Fig. 4)

3.1.3.2.2 Hepatic fibrosis was reversed by Chinese herb medicine

A little collagen fibers located only in portal areas or surrounded central veins in normal rat liver. Increased fibrous tissue formed thick interval that invaded into the hepatic lobules and moved round to form pseudolobules with different size in controls'liver. The fibrous intervals were thinner both in FZHY group and SA-B group than in controls. It means that hepatic fibrosis was reversed by FZHY recipe and SA-B. (Fig. 5)

3.1.3.2.3 The liver function of cirrhotic rats can be improved by Chinese herb medicine

Compared with normal rats, it was significantly increased in controls that are the activity of serum ALT and AST, serum level of TBiL (P<0.01 and P<0.05) but meanwhile the concentration of serum Alb were significantly decreased (P<0.05) . However, they were obviously lower both in FZHY group and SA-B group than in controls that are the activity of serum ALT and AST (P<0.01) , and serum level of TBiL (P<0.05) . The concentration of serum Alb were back to normal level with significantly difference compared with controls (P <0.05). (Fig. 6)

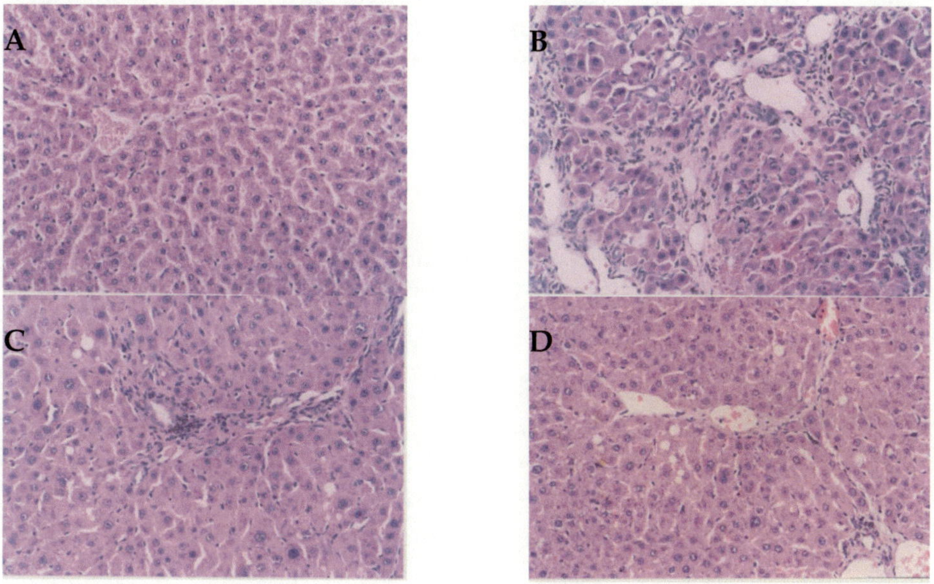

Fig. 4. Fuzheng Huayu Recipe and SA-B could relieve inflammation and structure damage in the liver tissue of DMN model rats A: normal group, B: control group, C: FZHY group and D: SA-B group. The staining was by HE (200×).

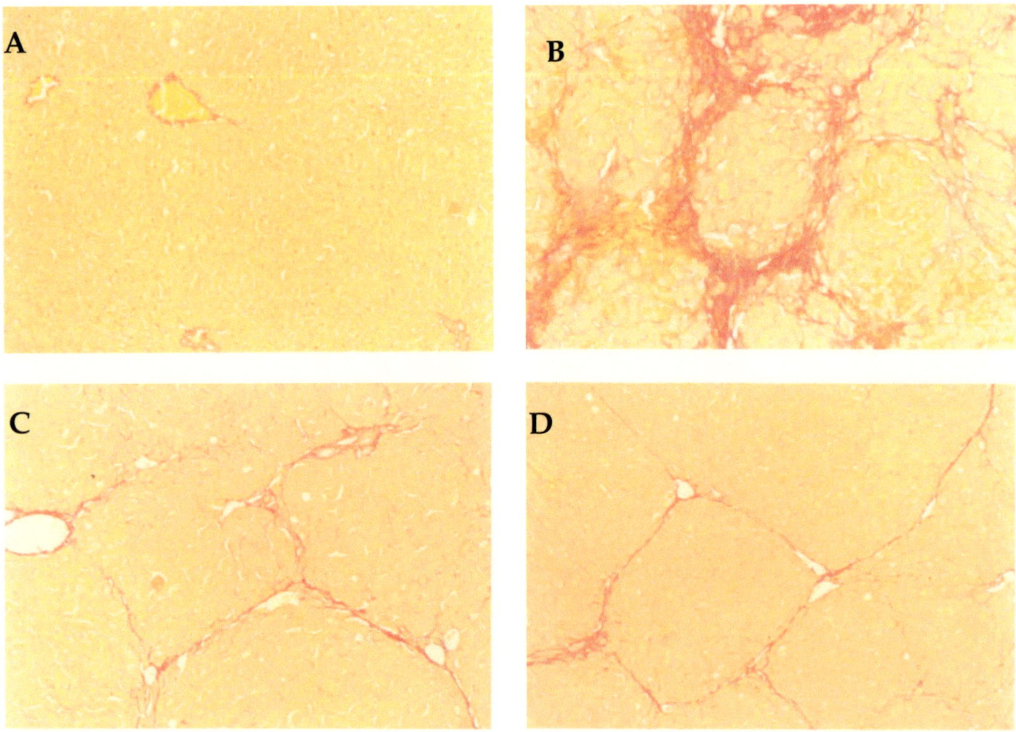

Fig. 5. Fuzheng Huayu Recipe and SA-B could relieve collagen fiber deposition in the liver tissue of DMN model rats A: normal group, B: control group, C: FZHY group, and D: SA-B group. The staining was by Sirius red (200×)

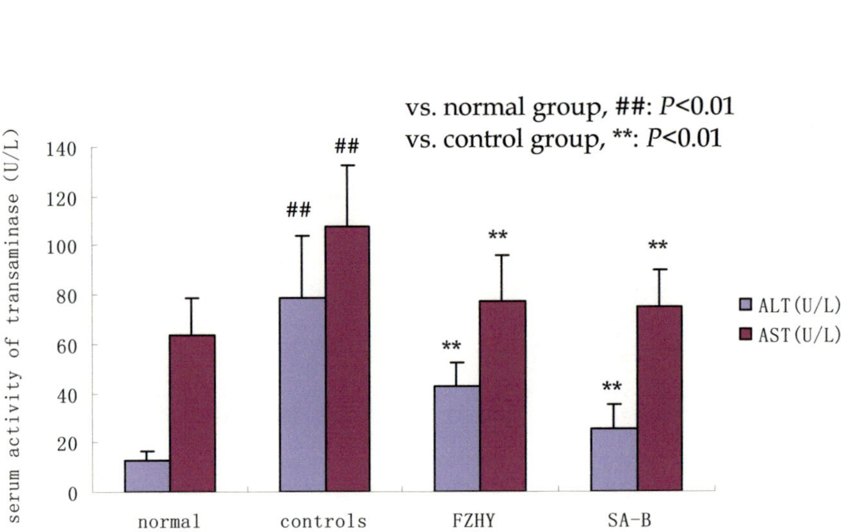

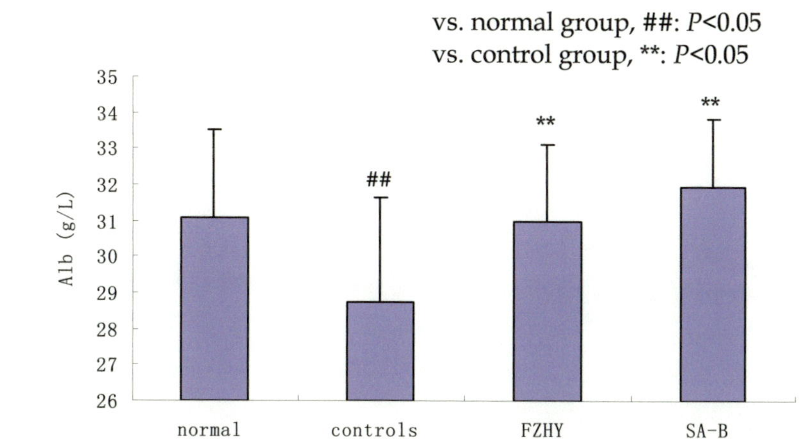

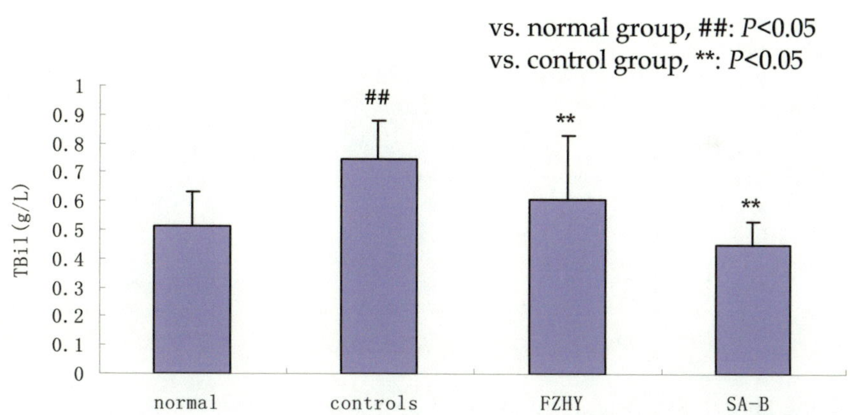

Fig. 6. Fuzheng Huayu Recipe and SA-B could decrease the avtivity of serum ALT and AST, and serum level of TBiL, but increase serum concentration of Alb in DMN model rats normal group, n=14; control group, n=9; FZHY group, n=13; SA-B group, n=14.

3.1.3.2.4 The concentration of Hyp in the liver tissue of cirrhotic rats was decreased by Chinese herb medicine

Compared with normal group, concentration of Hyp in the liver tissue was significantly increased at the end of experiment in controls ($P<0.01$). The concentration of Hyp, however, was significantly lower both in FZHY group and SA-B group than in controls ($P<0.05$). (Fig. 7)

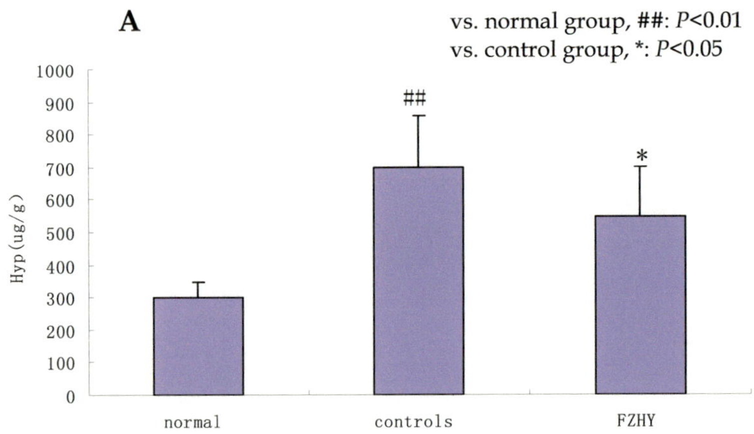

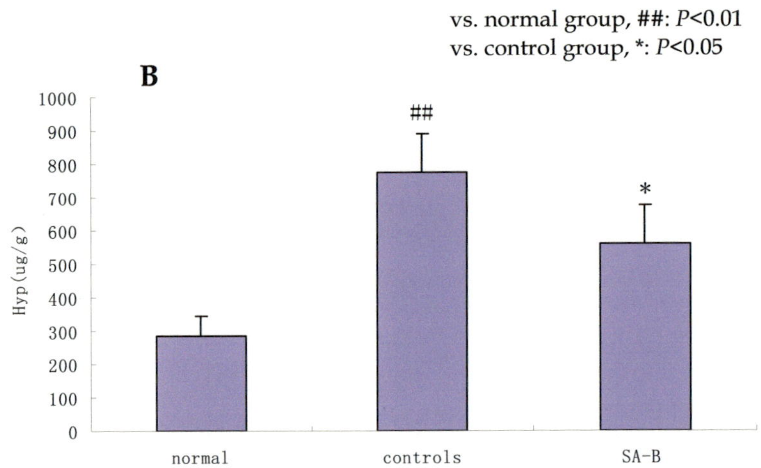

Fig. 7. Fuzheng Huayu Recipe and SA-B could decrease concentration of Hyp in the liver tissue of DMN model rats A. normal group, n=12; control group, n=9; FZHY group, n=12. B. normal group, n=13; control group, n=9; SA-B group, n=12.

3.1.3.2.5 Portal vein pressure of the cirrhotic rats was declined and the tissue concentration of ET-1 was dropped by Chinese herb medicine

The portal vein pressure of control rats was significantly increased in the end of experiment compared with normal rats (P<0.01). The increased range was up to 8mmHg. The portal pressure, however, was significantly lower in the rats treated with FZHY Recipe or SA-B than controls (P<0.05). (Fig. 8) The hepatic tissue concentration of ET-1 was obviously higher in controls than in normal group (P<0.01). But concentration of ET-1 was remarkably declined in FZHY group and SA-B group compared with controls (P<0.05). (Fig. 9.)

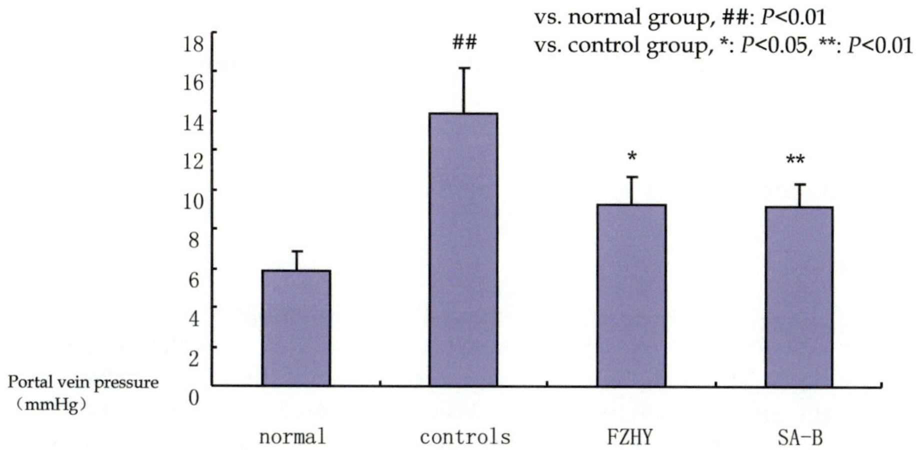

Fig. 8. Fuzheng Huayu Recipe and SA-B could decrease portal vein pressure in DMN model rats normal group, n=12; control group, n=9; FZHY group, n=13; SA-B group, n=14.

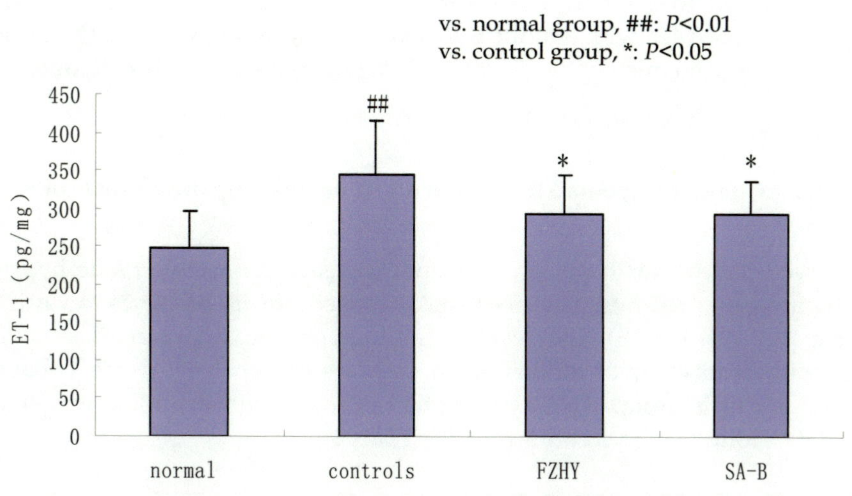

Fig. 9. Fuzheng Huayu Recipe and SA-B could decrease content of ET-1 in the liver tissue of DMN model rats normal group, n=14; control group, n=9; FZHY group, n=13; SA-B group, n=14.

3.1.4 Summary

The elevation of portal vein pressure is positively correlated with the increase of ET-1 concentration in the liver tissue during the process of liver cirrhosis. FZHY Recipe and SA-B can dramatically decrease the cirrhosis-induced elevation of portal vein pressure and concentration of ET-1 in the liver tissue through their effect on anti-fibrosis in the liver.

3.2 Experiment 2: Chinese herb medicine can relieve capillarization of sinusoid in cirrhotic rats

3.2.1 Aims

To investigate the effects of FZHY Recipe on capillarization of hepatic sinusoids.

3.2.2 Methods

32 Sprague-Dawley male rats, weighing about 150g, were randomly divided into normal group (n=7) and model group (n=25). The modeling mathod was the same as Experiment 1 for making cirrhosis. The cirrhotic rats were more randomly divided into control group (n=11), and FZHY group (n=14). The drug, dose and method of administration for each group were the same as Experiment 1, too. But the duration of treatment was for 4 weeks.

Rat's blood, under etherization condition, was collected from inferior vena cava, and was separated to serum. The sample of liver (1.0cm×0.8cm×0.3cm) was immediately taken and fixed in neutral formalin, embedded in paraffin, sectioned at 5 μm thick. The sections of liver were stained with HE, Masson and immunohistochemistry. Three rats were randomly selected from each group respectively for observation of hepatic microstructure. The each liver sample was cut to a 1 mm^3 cube, fixed with 2.5% glutaraldehyde and 1% osmium tetroxide for 2h, embedded with araldite 618, and cut to ultrathin sections. The sections were observed by the electron microscope (H-600). 100mg liver tissue was used to detect Hyp.

3.2.3 Results

3.2.3.1 Fuzheng Huayu Recipe had the potent effect against hepatic fibrosis of the model rat

It was observed that hemorrhage, necrosis and extensive connective tissue hyperplasia in the liver tissues of model rats. The fiber septa reached out its branches towards the liver lobule. (Fig. 10 and Tab. 3) The level of hydroxyproline was significantly increased. Compared with controls, liver inflammation, necrosis of hepatocytes and hepatic fibrosis was reduced in FZHY group. The concentration of liver hydroxyproline was significantly lower in FZHY group than in controls (*P*<0.05). (Tab. 4)

Groups	n	Hyperplasia degree of collagenous fibers				
		0	+	++	+++	++++
normal	7	7	0	0	0	0
controls	11	0	1	1	4	5
FZHY *	14	0	0	8	4	2

Note: compared with controls, *: U=4.06, *P*<0.01

Table 3. Hyperplasia degree of collagenous fibers in each group

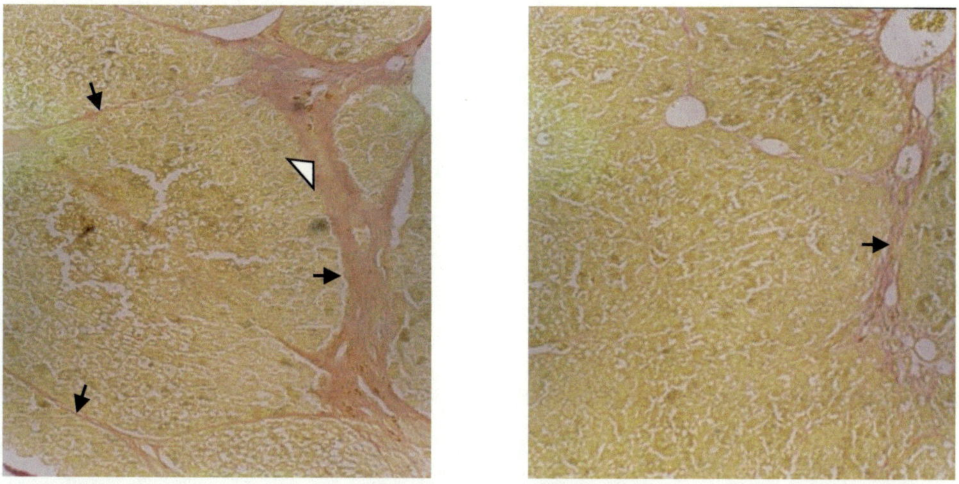

Fig. 10. Fuzheng Huayu Recipe inhibited hepatic fibrosis The liver sections were stained with Masson and showed hepatic fibrosis. A: Fibrous septa (arrows indicated) and pseudolobule (arrow's head indicated) have formed in controls. B: Fibrous septa (arrow indicated) is less and pseudolobule is absent in FZHY group (100×).

Groups	n	Hyp(μg/g liver wet weight)
normal	7	112.37±11.93
controls	11	292.83±36.78*
FZHY	14	215.03±75.46#

Note: compared with normal, *: $P<0.05$; compared with controls, #: $P<0.05$

Table 4. Liver Hydroxyproline level in liver tissues ($\bar{x}$ **±s**)

3.2.3.2 Fuzheng Huayu Recipe could effectively inhibit sinusoid capillarization in fibrotic rats

It was observed that the structure of sinusoids is clearly and the phenotype of SEC is thin by microscopy in normal group. There were many fenestrae in SEC cytoplasm and no basement membrane covered on SEC in perisinusoid side. In controls, the sinusoids were twisted and narrow, the fenestrae in SEC were reduced or disappeared, and basement membrane was observed. (Fig.11)Factor Ⅷ related antigen (Ⅷ R·Ag), α-smooth muscle actin (α-SMA) and laminin (LM), the important indexes for hepatic sinusoid capillarization, were positive staining in liver tissure. But collagen type Ⅳ (Col Ⅳ), which is a composition of functional membrane but not a composition of basement membrane, expressed majorly in fibrous septa and HSC but less and discontinuously in perisinusoids in controls. Compared with controls, however, the narrow sinusoids were reduced and some sinusoids returned to normal phenotype, basement membrane looked discontinuous thiner, and the positive degree of Ⅷ R·Ag, α-SMA and LM were lower and their positive area was significantly smaller by image analysis in the liver of FZHY group than in that of controls ($P<0.05$). Col Ⅳ expressed still continuously in perisinusoids in FZHY group. It indicated that the normal structure of sinusoids was most kept and it meansed that the alteration of hepatic sinusoid capillarization was reversed. (Fig.12)

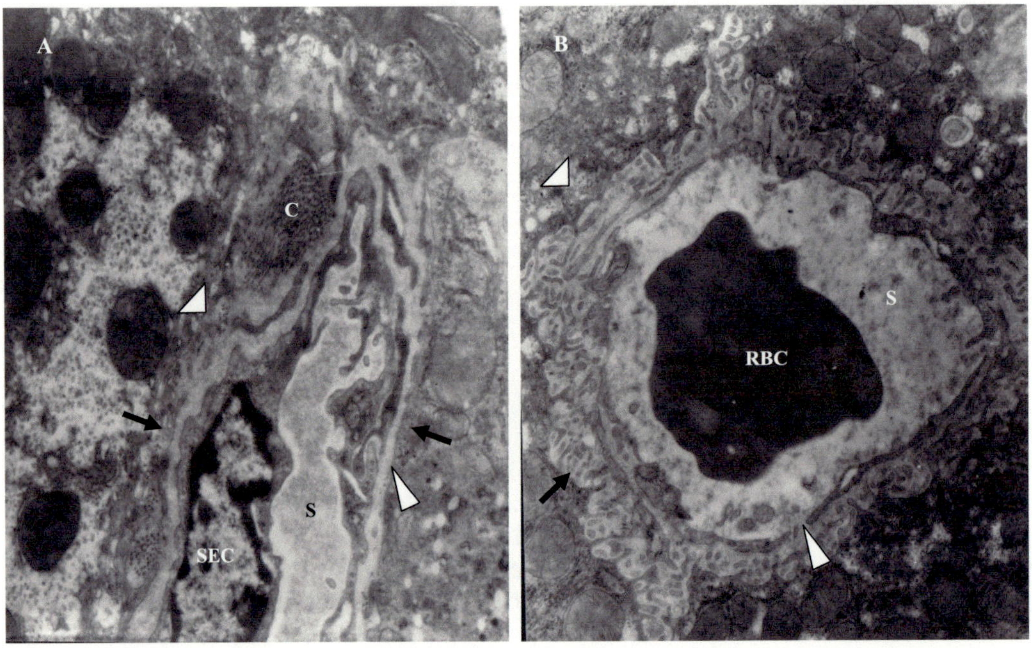

Fig. 11. Fuzheng Huayu Recipe could inhibit sinusoid capillarization by observation of electron micrographs S: sinusoid; C: collagen. A: Hepatic sinusoid appeare as a typical capillary surrounded by continuous basement membrane. (arrow's heads indicated) in the liver of fibrotic rat. The perisinusoid is stenosis (arrows indicated) and microvilli of hepatocyte are almost absent in the space (15000×). B: Sinusoid capillarization is not formed in the liver of rat treated with Fuzheng Huayu Recipe. The fenestrae are observed (arrow's heads indicated) in cytoplasm of SEC. A mass of microvilli of hepatocyte stretchs into perisinusoid is exist (arrow indicated) but basement membrane is absent (10000×).

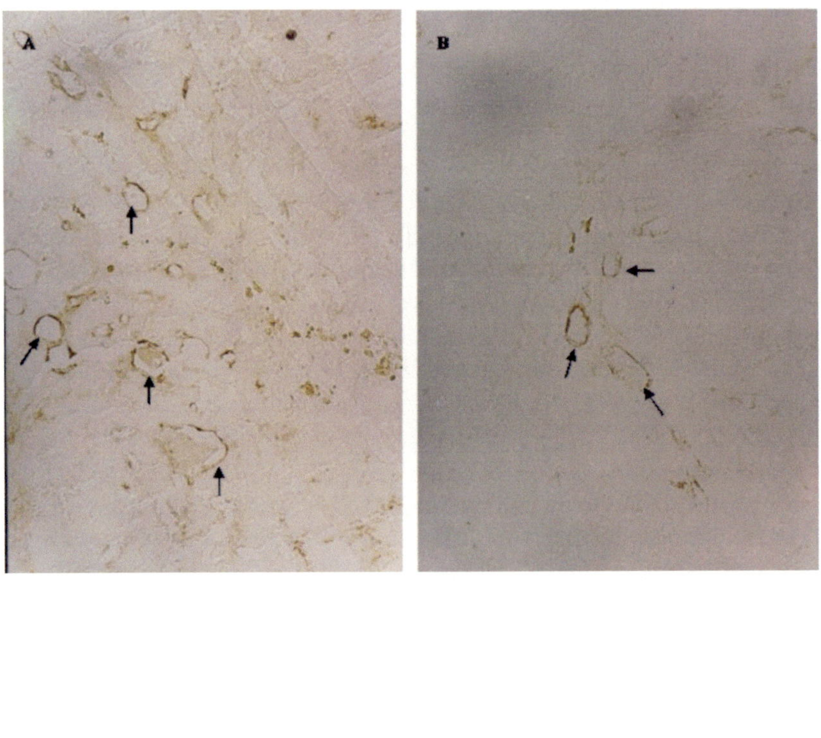

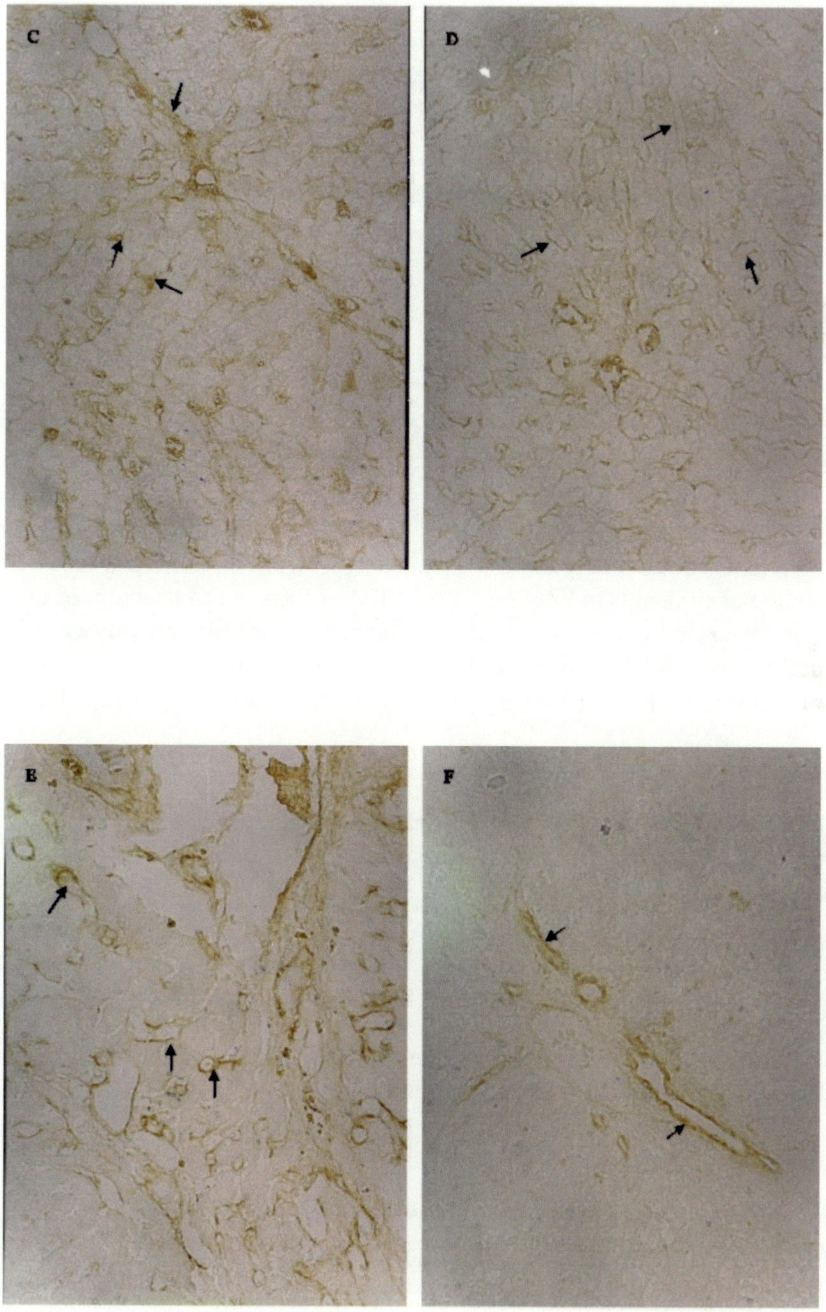
C
D
E
F

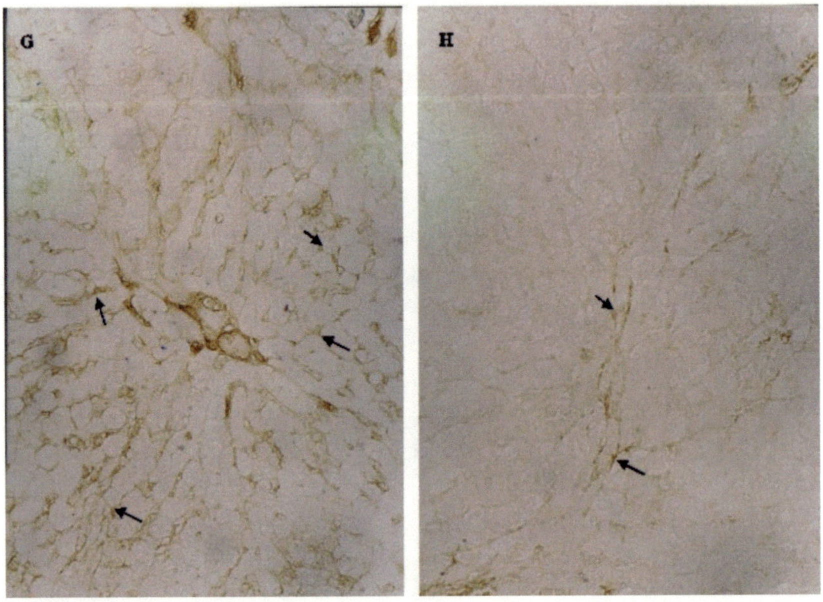

Fig. 12. Fuzheng Huayu Recipe could alter the express of indexes for hepatic sinusoid capillarization by immunohistochemistry staining in fibrotic liver of rats Arrows show the positive area. A: Ⅷ R·Ag is around the vessels with strong staining in controls. B: The positive area of Ⅷ R·Ag is decreased in FZHY group. C: Col IV expresses majorly in fibrous septa and HSC but less and discontinuously in perisinusoids in controls. D: Col IV expresses almost continuously in perisinusoids in FZHY group. E: The express of LM is observed on the wall of vessels and sinusoids in the liver of controls. F: The express of LM is only observed on the wall of vessels in the liver of FZHY group. G: α-SMA expresses strongly in perisinusoids, HSC and fibous septa in controls. H: α-SMA expresses dramaticlly less in FZHY group (100×).

3.2.4 Summary

Fuzheng Huayu Recipe had the potent effect on against liver fibrosis. The one of mechanisms of the recipe perhaps is associated with inhibition of hepatic sinusoid capillarization.

3.3 Experiment 3: SA-B could decrease portal vein pressure in rats induced by ET-1

3.3.1 Aims

To establish a rat model of portal hypertension induced by ET-1 and investigate the effect of SA-B on decreasing portal vein pressure in the model.

3.3.2 Methods

3.3.2.1 To establish portal hypertension model of rats induced by ET-1

48 Sprague-Dawley male rats were randomly divided into four groups: the NS solution group, the ET-1 low-dose group (0.3μg/kg body weight), the ET-1 medium-dose group

(1.0μg/kg body weight) and the ET-1 high-dose group (3.0μg/kg body weight). Rats were injected with 200μl NS solution into rat via femoral vein by a pump with a rate of 80μl/min in NS solution group. As the same method, rats were injected with 200ml ET-1 solution with the dose of 0.3μg/kg body weight, 1.0μg/kg body weight or 3.0μg/kg body weight respectively in 3 ET-1 groups. Then, monitored the changes of carotid pressure and portal vein pressure in each group at 2min, 4min, 6min, 8min, 10min, 15min, 20min, 25min and 30min after injection.

3.3.2.2 To treat rats with drugs in portal hypertension models

20 Sprague-Dawley male rats with about 330g body weight were randomly divided into four groups: normal group, SA-B group, BQ-123 (ET_AR antagonist) group and BQ-788 (ET_BR antagonist) group (n=5 in each group). In normal group, BQ-123 group and BQ-788 group, rats were gavaged with water at a dose of 1ml/100g body weight and rats in SA-B group were gavaged with SA-B solution (containing 125mg/100ml) at the same dose. The gavage was performed twice per day for 5 days. The experiment started at 1 hour after the final gavage. First, via rat's femoral vein, rats was injected with BQ-123 (12.5μg/kg body weight) in BQ-123 group and with BQ-788 (15μg/kg body weight) in BQ-788 group. 30min later, rats were injected with a dose (3μg/kg body weight) of ET-1 solution by a pump with rate of 80μl/min in each group. Then, the portal vein pressure was measured before and after injection of ET-1.

3.3.2.3 To measure carotid pressure, heart rate and portal vein pressure

A piece of PE-50 tube, which full with heparin solution, was inserted into the left carotid artery of the rat. Following that, connect the tube to a pressure transducer in order to measure carotid pressure and heart rate. Then a piece of PE-10 tube, which full with heparin solution, was inserted from superior mesenteric vein to the middle of portal vein. Connect the tube to a pressure transducer for measurement of portal vein pressure.

3.3.3 Results

3.3.3.1 A kind of model of rat with portal hypertension was successfully established by injection of ET-1

There was no obvious effect of solution volume on carotid pressure and portal vein pressure after injection of NS solution. ET-1 solution with equal volume of NS solution was injected into the rats in low- and medium-dose groups. The carotid pressure was not noticeable rise or fall, only minor fluctuations within 20 min after injection. The carotid pressure, however, was increased slightly after injection of ET-1 in high-dose group but the alteration was not significant (Fig.13). Portal vein pressure was increased in short time after injection of ET-1 although the alteration was not same in three different dose groups. The alteration of pressure was most remarkable in high-dose group than in others. After reaching to peak level, portal vein pressure was stable for 4min, 4min and 10min in low-, medium- and high-dose groups, respectively (Fig.14 and Tab. 5). The results indicated that the increase of portal vein pressure was solely caused by the injection of ET-1 and without related with the volume of solution in this kind of animal model. This inducing method would not cause a significant increase of systemic blood pressure. Compared with the existing portal vein perfusion model, this kind of portal hypertension model is more similar to the "living" state. It was also avoided that increase of portal vein pressure caused by sudden increase of partial blood volume by quickly direct injection of ET-1 in portal vein. This kind of model would better reflect the true effect of ET-1 compared with other kind of model. Therefore, this kind of model could use not only for investigation of efficacy and mechanism of drug, but also provided an ideal experimental subject for screening drugs to treat portal hypertension.

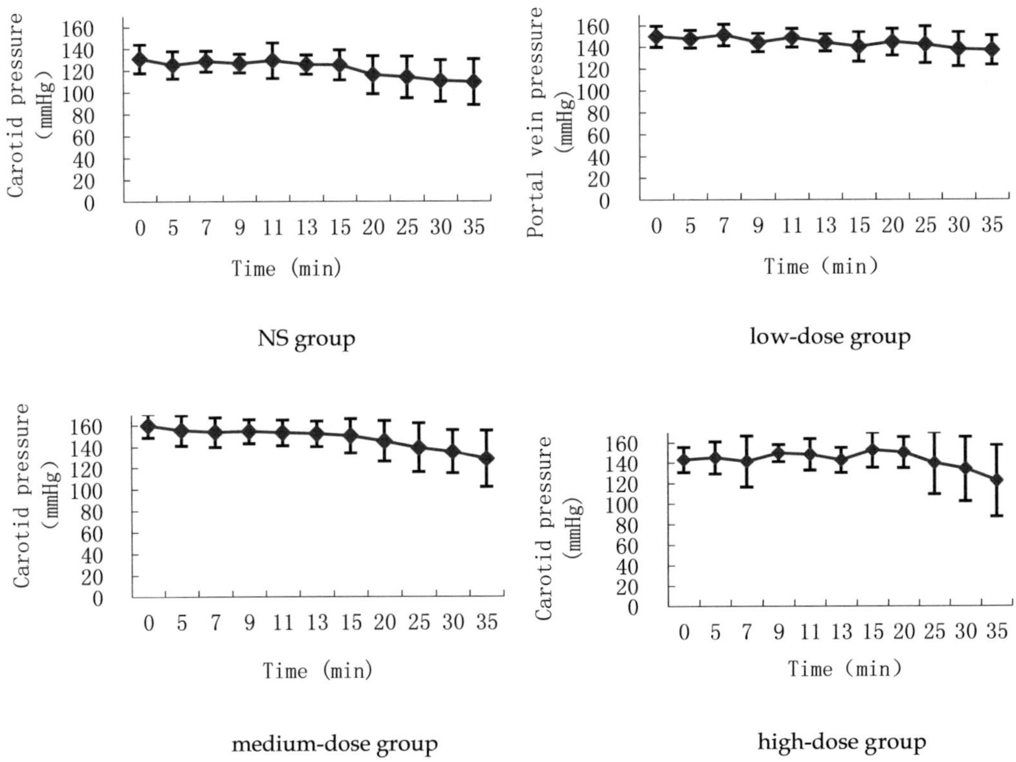

Fig. 13. Effect of ET-1 with different doses on rat carotid pressures After detecting carotic pressure for 5min, NS solution or ET-1 with same volume but different doses were constantly injected and carotic pressure was detected for 30min. The pressure was not increased during detected time in NS group, and low- and medium-dose groups. But the carotid pressure was increased slightly in high-dose group.

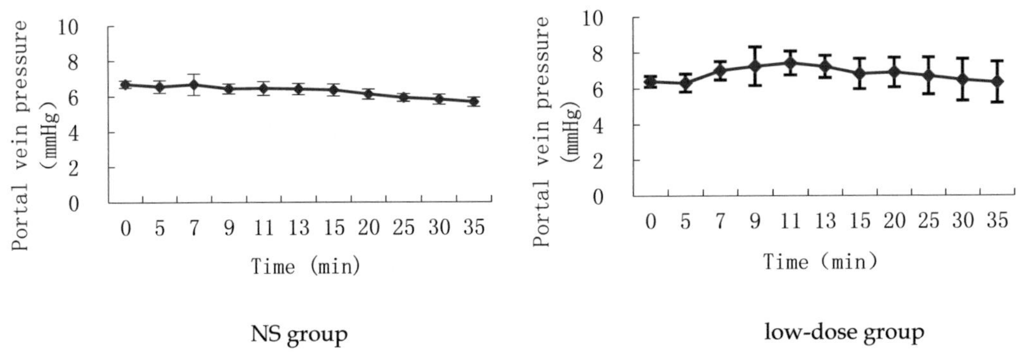

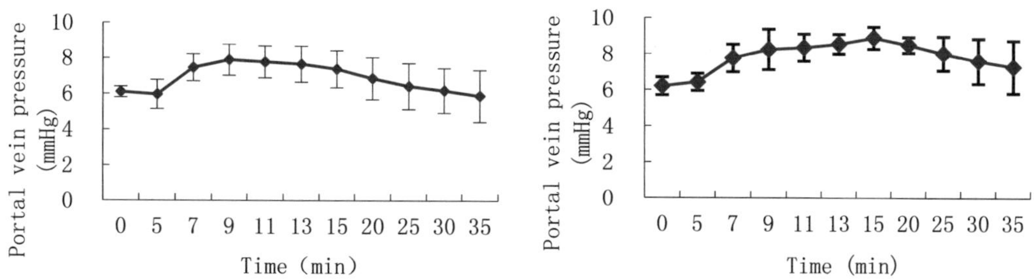

medium-dose group high-dose group

Fig. 14. Effect of ET-1 with different doses on rat portal vein pressure After detecting portal vein pressure for 5min, NS solution and ET-1 with same volume but different doses were constantly injected and portal vein pressure was detected for 30min. There was no obvious effect of NS solution on portal vein pressure. The pressure was increased at 5min when starting injection of ET-1 and kept high level for 4min, 4min and 10min in low-, medium- and high-dose groups after the pressure reaching to a peak level at 9 min, respectively.

Groups	n	Initial pressure	Highest pressure	Increased range
		(mmHg)	(mmHg)	(mmHg)
NS	8	6.6±0.3	6.5±0.4	-0.1±0.2
low-dose	10	6.1±0.8	7.5±0.8**	1.3±0.3▲▲▲
medium-dose	10	6.3±0.5	8.1±0.6**	1.8±0.5▲▲▲##
high-dose	9	6.0±0.6	8.5±0.9**	2.5±0.5▲▲▲##☆☆

Note: compared with the initial pressure in the interior-group, **: *P*<0.01; compared with NS group, ▲▲▲: *P*<0.001; compared with low-dose group, ##: *P*<0.01; compared with medium-dose group, ☆☆: *P*<0.01

Table 5. Effect of ET-1 with different doses on portal vein pressure of rats ($\bar{X}$±S)

Groups	n	Initial pressure	Highest pressure	Increased range
		(mmHg)	(mmHg)	(mmHg)
control	5	6.1±0.7	8.6±1.1***	2.5±0.4
SA-B	5	6.1±0.7	7.8±1.6**	1.6±0.5##
BQ-123	5	5.9±1.1	7.1±1.0	1.2±0.2###
BQ-788	5	5.9±0.9	6.9±1.1	0.98±0.5###

Note: compared with initial pressure interior-group, **: *P*<0.01, ***: *P*<0.001; compared with the controls, ##: *P*<0.01, ###: *P*<0.001

Table 6. Effect of SA-B, BQ-123 or BQ-788 on reducining portal vein pressure of rats induced by ET-1 ($\bar{X}$±S)

3.3.3.2 SA-B could inhibit the rise of portal vein pressure in rats induced by ET-1

Portal vein pressur significantly increased after ET-1 solution (3μg/kg body weight) was injected to rats pretreated with water by gavage. Although portal vein pressure of the rats, which were pretreated with SA-B solution by gavage or with BQ-123 or BQ-788 by injection, was also increased after ET-1 injection, however, the ranget-increased was obviously less than that in controls (*P*<0.01, *P*<0.001) (Tab.6). Furthermore, the stable time, when portal vein pressure kept high level after reaching peak level, was short in SA-B group. It was just 6 min in SA-B group but was 10min in controls. (Fig. 15)

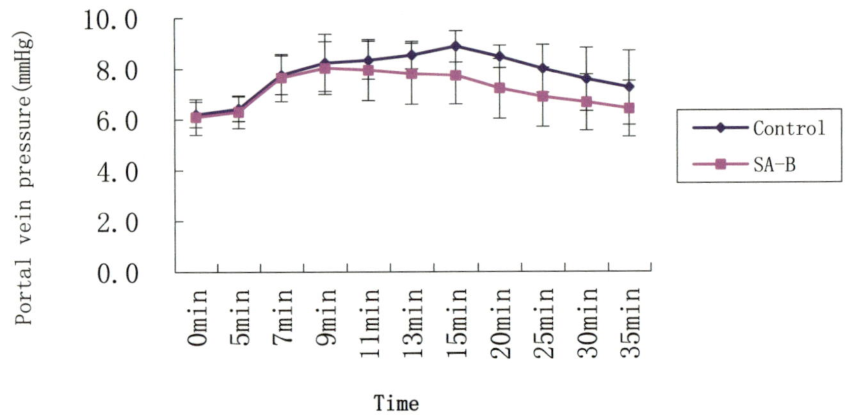

Fig. 15. SA-B could inhibit portal vein pressure of rats induced by ET-1 Portal vein pressure began increase at 5min when starting injection of ET-1. The peak level of pressure was at 9min in SA-B group. Then the pressure kept high level until to at 15min. In controls, however, the pressure continuously increased until to highest peak level at 15min and began to decrease. The pressure level was still hinger (a little bit higher than a peak level in SA-B group) until to at 25min.

Groups	n	Carotid artery pressure	Heart rate
		(mmHg)	(Beats/min)
control	3	130.9±13.2	439±21
SA-B	5	145.6±10.1	439±21

Table 7. Compare of the carotid artery pressure and heart rate in SA-B group and controls

3.3.3.3 SA-B did not affect on carotid pressure and heart rate in normal rat

Rats were pretreated with SA-B solution by gavage for 5d, but the carotid pressure and heart rate were no significant different between in SA-B group and controls. (Tab.7)

3.3.4 Summary

A kind of rat model of portal hypertension is successfully established by injection of ET-1. SA-B can down regulate the raised portal vein pressure by antagonizing the effect of extraneous ET-1.

3.4 Experiment 4: SA-B can decrease portal vein pressure in mice induced by ET-1

3.4.1 Aims

To establish portal hypertension model of mice induced by ET-1 and investigate the effect of SA-B on decreasing portal vein pressure in this kind of model.

3.4.2 Methods

3.4.2.1 To establish a kind of portal hypertension model mice induced by ET-1

36 male Kunming mices, 30±5g body weight, were randomly divided into three groups: control group (n=12), SA-B group (n=12) and blocker group (n=12). Mice were gavaged with SA-B (1mg/ml) in SA-B group and gavaged with water in control group and blocker group. The volume of gvage was 0.5 ml per mouse once a day for 3days. Mice were injected with BQ-123 (2μg/kg body weight) by tail vein at 0.5h before start of below experiment in blocker group.

Mice were injected with ET-1 (1.6μg/kg body weight) at constant velocity by tail vein. 6 mice were randomly taken out from each group to measure blood flow volume in liver microcirculation using a laser-Doppler flow instrument before and after injection of ET-1. Other 6 mice in each group were measured the blood flow rate in liver microcirculation by an inverted fluorescence microscope with microscopic live video technology before and after injection of ET-1.

3.4.2.2 To measure the average blood flow volume in the perfusion of liver microcirculation

Each mouse was injected with 2% pentobarbital sodium solution at a dose of 2ml/kg body weight for anesthesia. After opening abdomen the liver was put on a detector connected with a laser-Doppler flow instrument to record the blood flow volum in the perfusion of liver microcirculation for 5min. After a pause, ET-1 was injected by a syringe pump at a constant rate of 80μl/ min through tail vein. Then, the blood flow volum was recorded again for 5min. The average blood flow volume was calculated from the stable datas during the former 5min record and late 5min record, respectively.

3.4.2.3 To measure the blood flow rate in liver microcirculation

Each mouse was injected with 2% pentobarbital sodium solution at a dose of 2ml/kg body weight for anesthesia. After opening abdomen the liver was put on a piece of glass plate which was on an inverted fluorescence microscope. After 0.05ml pre-labeled erythrocytes with FITC was injected into the inferior vena cava, a suitable site was focused to observe the liver microcirculation. Some FITC-RBCs were observed to be moving quickly in microvasculature or sinusoids and recorded with digital video. ET-1(1.6μg /kg body weight) was injected by a syringe pump at a constant rate of 80μl/ min through tail vein of mouse then moving FITC-RBCs were immediately recorded again with digital video. The moving range of FITC-RBCs in record was calculated by the analytic software to compare the differences of blood flow rate in liver microcirculation in 3 groups.

3.4.3 Results

3.4.3.1 SA-B reduced average blood flow volume in liver microcirculation

The blood flow volume in liver microcirculation was decreased in 3 groups after injection of ET-1. The reduced range was smaller in SA-B group and in block group than in controls ($P<0.01$). (Tab. 8)

3.4.3.2 SA-B reduced average blood flow rate in liver microcirculation

The blood flow rate in liver microcirculation was significantly decreased after injection of ET-1 ($P<0.01$). But the reduced range was smaller in SA-B group and in blocker group than in controls ($P<0.05$ and $P<0.01$). (Tab. 9)

Average blood flow volume in liver microcirculation (BPU)				
Groups	**n**	**Before ET-1 injection**	**After ET-1 injection**	**Reduced range**
control	6	1186.83±41.14	1060.50±18.33	126.33±27.51
SA-B	6	1269.50±59.90	1189.33±40.33	80.17±20.30 **
blocker	6	202.00±36.54	1131.00±23.67	71.00±12.82 **

Note: compared with the controls, **: $P<0.01$

Table 8. SA-B and BQ-123 could inhibit reduction of average blood flow volume in mice induced by ET-1 ($\bar{X} \pm S$)

Blood flow rate in liver microcirculation (mm/s)				
Groups	**n**	**Before ET-1 injection**	**After ET-1 injection**	**Reduced range**
Control	6	0.60±0.01	0.36±0.02☆☆	0.23±0.02
SA-B	6	0.62±0.04	0.39±0.01☆☆	0.18±0.04 *
blocker	6	0.60±0.05	0.43±0.01☆☆	0.17±0.05 **

Note: compared with initial blood flow rate,☆☆: $P<0.01$; compared with controls, *: $P<0.05$, **: $P<0.01$

Table 9. SA-B and BQ-123 could inhibit reduction of the liver blood flow rate in mice induced by ET-1 ($\bar{X} \pm S$).

3.4.4 Summary

The average blood flow volume and blood flow rate in mice liver microcirculation were reduced by extraneous ET-1. SA-B could inhibit the effect of ET-1 to improve liver microcirculation.

4. The experiment *in vitro*

It is believed that recipe of herb medicine is not suitable for research of mechanism *in vitro*. For more studying the mechanism of Fuzheng Huayu Recipe on reducing portal hypertension, we can only select SA-B as investigated subject *in vitro*.

4.1 Aims

To investigate the effects of SA-B on inhibiting contraction of human HSC induced by ET-1.

4.2 Methods

4.2.1 To observe contraction of HSC

Human HSC was isolated from the normal section of transplant patients'liver by enzymatic digestion and density-gradient centrifugation with Nycodenz solution.[14]. Passaged HSC was planted on the collagen gel which was pre-poured into 12-wells plates. After cells had adhered, HSC was divided into 5 groups: 1) serum-free group in which HSC was cultured with serum-free M199; 2) ET group in which HSC was treated with ET-1(10^{-8} mol/L); 3) low-dose group in which HSC was treated with ET-1 and 10^{-7}mol/L SA-B; 4) medium-dose group in which HSC was treated with ET-1 and 10^{-6}mol/L SA-B; 5) high-dose group in which HSC was treated with ET-1 and 10^{-5}mol/L SA-B._The edge of the gel was scraped out wall of the well by a syringe needle after adding drugs. The diameter of gel was observed at 2h, 4h, 6h, and 12 h during HSC culture and a gel image analysis system was used to calculate the area of gel. The area of gel can indicate the contractibility of HSC. The experiment was repeated for 3 times.

4.2.2 To detect the concentration of free calcium ([Ca^{2+}]i) in HSC

HSC was planted in 6-wells plates. Flu-3/AM was added into media with final concentration of 5μmol/L. Then HSC was in a incubator with 37°C, 5%CO_2-95% humid air and dark for 30min. HSC was washed twice with serum-free M199 for moving the dye and divided into 5 groups as above. HSC in each group was observed under a laser confocal microscope before and after adding relevant drugs. The observation conditions were Kr/Ar laser, excitation wavelength 488nm, emission wavelength 505-530nm. The experiment was repeated 2 times.

4.3 Results

4.3.1 SA-B inhibited contraction of HSC induced by ET-1

Area of gel was significantly bigger in low-dose group (2209.02±177.96μm^2), medium-dose group (2164.95±111.84μm^2) and high-dose group (2374.73±218.38μm^2) than in ET group (156.23±102.16μm^2). The statistical difference was dramatically (P<0.01). But there was no obviously difference among in 3 SA-B treatment groups. (Fig. 16)_The morphological changes of HSC showed dose-dependent after incubation with SA-B. The phenotype of HSC in low-dose group was similar to that in ET group. The phenotype of HSC in high-dose group was similar to that in serum-free group. The phenotype of HSC in medium-dose group was between the low- and high-dose groups. (Fig. 17)

4.3.2 SA-B suppressed the intracellular concentration of [Ca^{2+}]i in HSC induced by ET-1

Compared with ET group in which fluorescence of HSC was very strong, [Ca^{2+}]i fluorescence image appeared the opposite phenomenon in 3 SA-B treatment groups. Only a few cells appeared slightly enhanced fluorescent and the intracellular concentration of

$[Ca^{2+}]i$ was obviously lower in 3 SA-B treatment groups than in ET group. The intracellular concentration of $[Ca^{2+}]i$ was weak and only two relative low-lying peaks were in low-dose group within 120sec. The alteration of intracellular concentration of $[Ca^{2+}]i$ was smaller in medium-dose group and high-dose group during observation. (Fig.18). The results indicated that one of mechanisms of SA-B on inhibiting contraction of HSC may be related with that SA-B suppressed the intracellular concentration of $[Ca^{2+}]i$ in HSC.

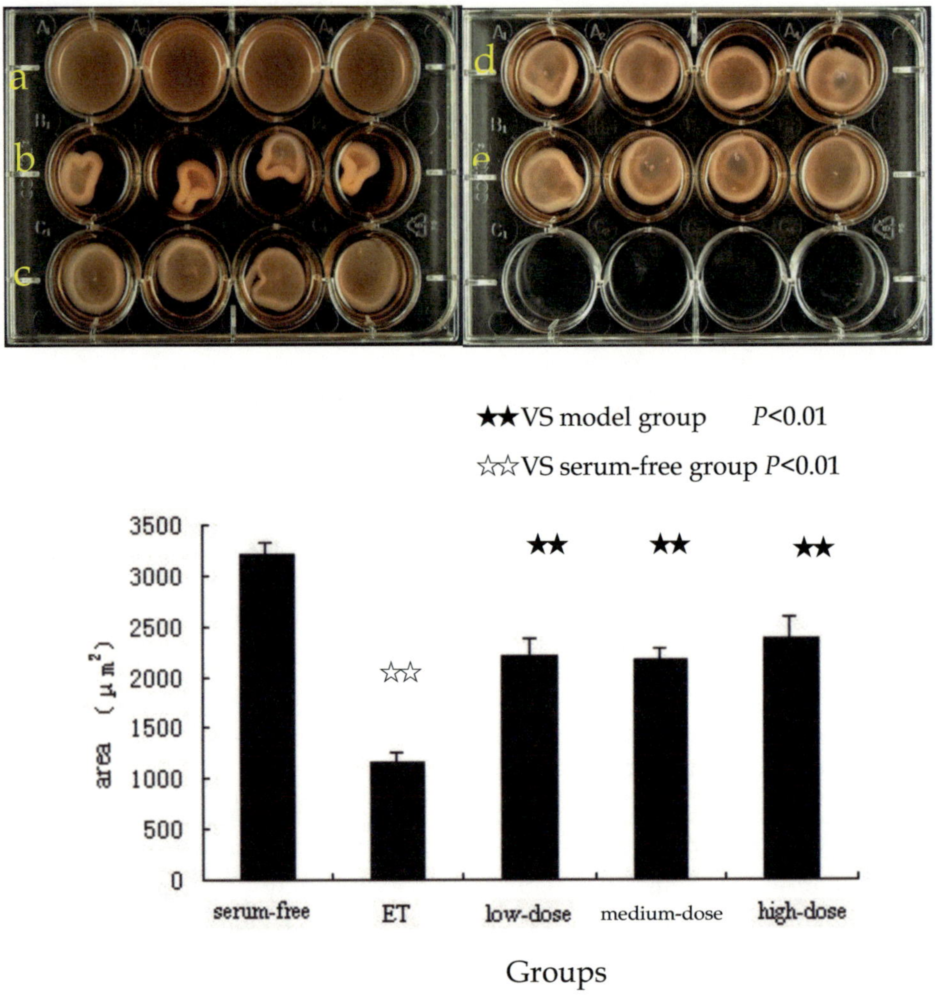

Fig. 16. SA-B could inhibit contraction of human HSC a: serum-free group; b: ET group; c: low-dose group; d: medium-dose group; e: high-dose group. Human HSC was cultured on collangen gel. Actived HSC are able to contract to lead to area of gel becoming small. In serum-free group, contraction capacity of HSC was weak so that the area of gel was nearly invariant. Active HSC induced by ET-1 contracted strongly. The area of gel was significantly smaller in ET group than in serum-free groups. SA-B could inhibit contraction of HSC induced by ET-1. The area of gel was bigger in 3 SA-B treatment groups than in ET group.

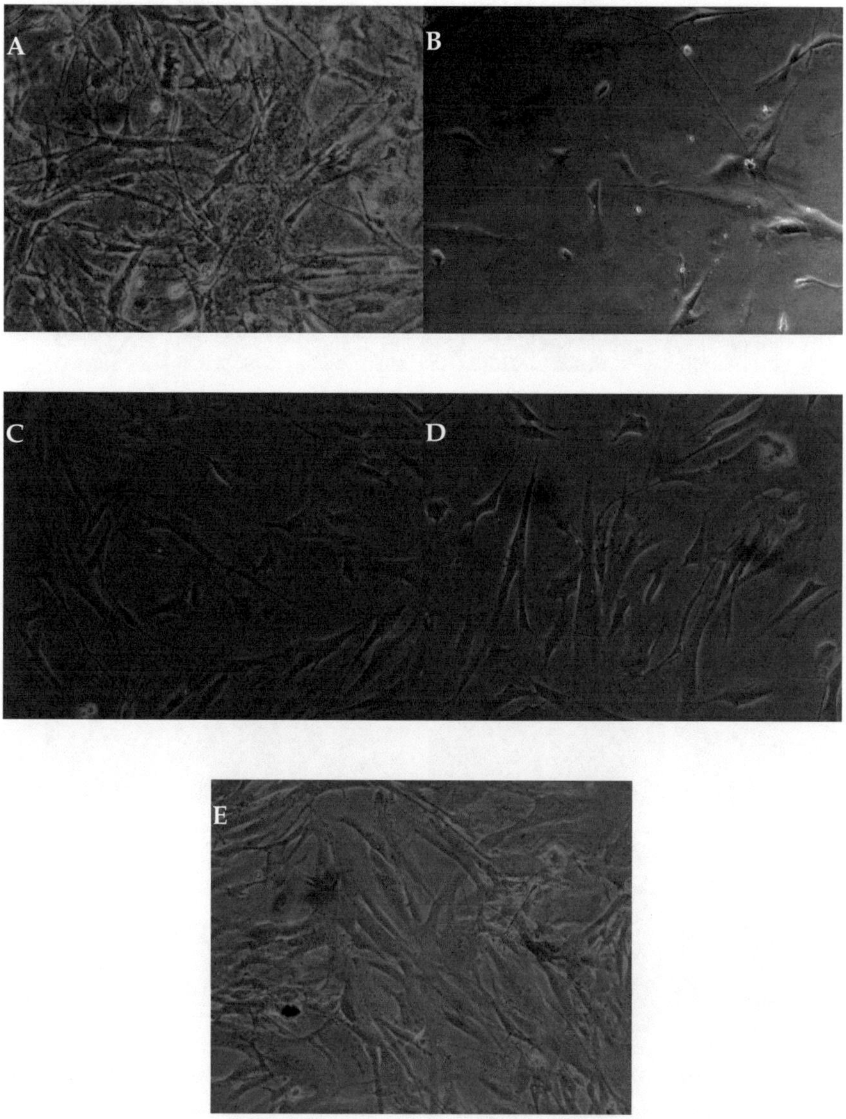

Fig. 17. The morphological changes of HSC in each group a: serum-free group; b: ET group; c: low-dose group; d: medium-dose group; e: high-dose group. HSC grew exuberantly on gel and the pseudopodium of HSC was a lot, thin and long in serum-free group. After induced by ET-1 for 12h, however, HSC became obviously small with contraction. The quantity and the pseudopodium of HSC was decreased in ET group. The phenotype of HSC in low-dose group was similar to that in ET group. The phenotype of HSC in high-dose group was similar to that in serum-free group. The phenotype of HSC in medium-dose group was between the low- and high-dose groups (By OLYMPUS I × 50 / I × 70 inverted system microscope, Japan, 200×).

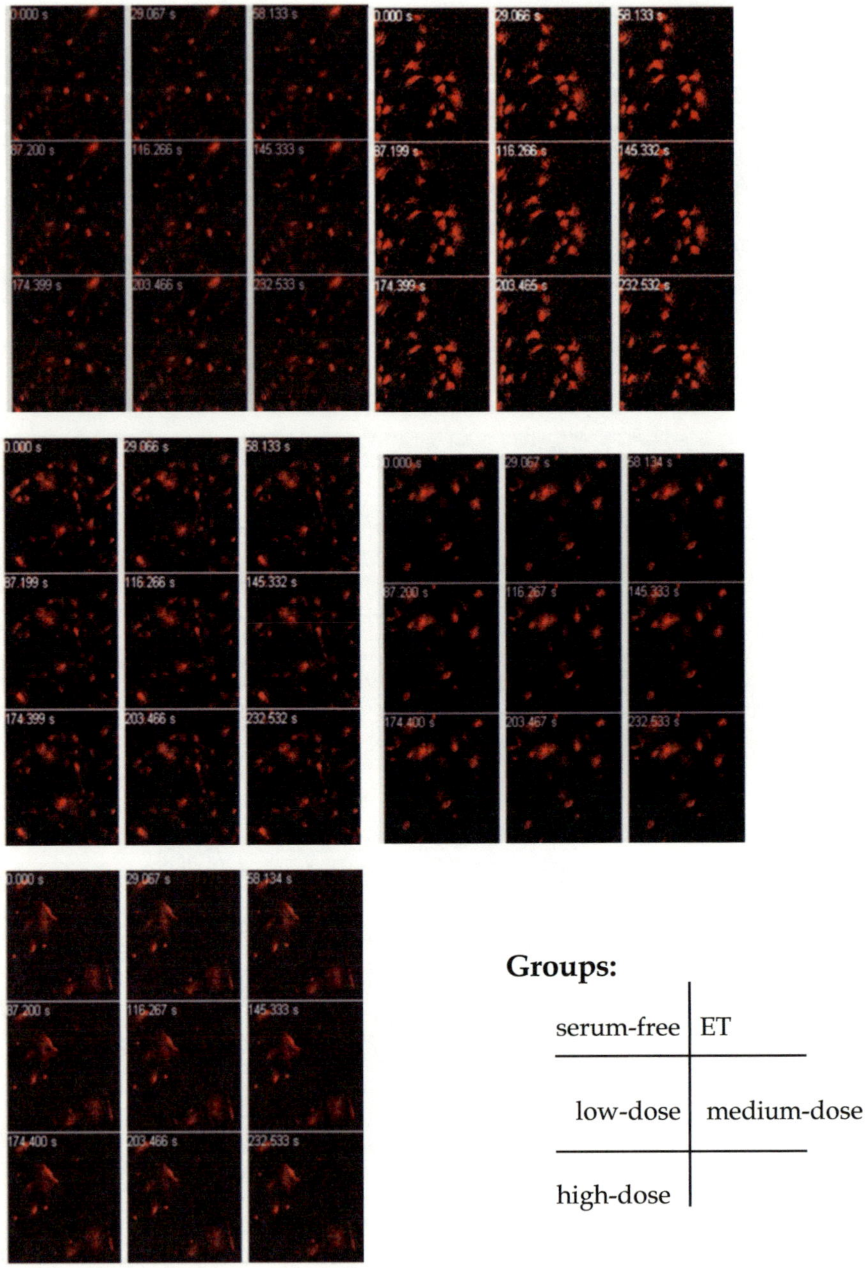

Fig. 18. SA-B suppressed the intracellular concentration of $[Ca^{2+}]i$ in HSC Fluorescent of Flu-3/AM which represents the intracellular concentration of $[Ca^{2+}]i$ was observed. The expression of fluorescent in HSC was very stronger in ET group than in serum-free group. But the expression of fluoresent in HSC was dose-dependent in 3 SA-B treatment groups. The higher the dose of SA-B was, the weaker expression of fluorescent was (By Zeiss510 laser confocal microscope, German, 200×).

5. Conclusion

The Chinese medicine, Fuzheng Huayu Recipe, is able to reduce portal hypertension in liver cirrhosis both in clinic and *in vivo*. The effect of Fuzheng Huayu Recipe is related with reversing hepatic fibrosis and capillarization, and decreasing concentration of ET-1 in the liver tissue. SA-B is an extracted component of Fuzheng Huayu Recipe. Several studies showed that the effect in SA-B was similar to Fuzheng Huayu Recipe on reversing hepatic fibrosis and decreasing concentration of ET-1 in the liver tissue. SA-B inhibited contraction of HSC through suppressing the intracellular concentration of $[Ca^{2+}]i$. Based on above effects, intrahepatic vessel resistance was reduced which leaded to improve liver microcirculation. It has distinctively character that Chinese herb medicine is used to treat hepatic portal hypertension which is caused by failure of liver microcirculation in chronic liver diseases.

6. Acknowledgements

This work was supported by grants from National Natural Science Foundation of China 30672489; Leading Academic Discipline Project of Shanghai Municipal Education Commission J50307; E-Institute of TCM Internal Medicine, Shanghai Municipal Education Commission E03008; Innovation Research Team in Universities, Shanghai Municipal Education Commission; and Leading Academic Discipline Project of Hepatology, SATCM (2011sh). Translation assistance from Lu Chao, Wang Meifeng, Zhang Jing, Wu Mei and Pan Yuanwei is gratefully acknowledged.

7. Reference

McCuskey RS. The hepatic microvascular system in health and its response to toxicants. Anat Rec (Hoboken). 2008,291(6):661-71.

Wu Zhiyong. Regulation of liver microcirculation and portal hypertension. J. Hepatopancreatobiliary Surgery. 2000,12(1):53-54.

Pinzani M, Milani S, Defranco R, et al. Endothelin 1 is overexpressed in human cirrhotic liver and exerts multiple effects on activated hepatic stellate cells. Gastroenterology 1996,110:534-548.

Vollmar B, Menger. The hepatic microcirculation: mechanistic contributions and therapeutic targets in liver injury and repair. Physiol Rev. 2009,89(4):1269-339.

Spengler U. Hepatic microcirculation: a critical but neglected factor for the outcome of viral hepatitis. J Hepatol. 2009,50(3):631-3.

Nishida J, McCuskey RS, McDonnell D. Protective Role of NO in Hepatic Microcirculatory Dysfunction during Endotoxemia. Am J Physiol. 1994,267(6 Pt 1):G1135-41.

Ramadori G. The stellate cell of the liver. Virchows Arch B Cell Pathol 1991, 61:147-158.

Pinzani M. Hepatic stellate (ITO) cells: expanding roles for a liver-specific pericyte. J Hepatol 1995, 22: 700-706.

ZHANG Jie, XU Lieming, ZHANG Wenwei. Study of Effect and Mechanism of Salvianolic-acid B Salt on Inhibiting the Contraction of Human Hepatic Stellate Cells Induced by Endothelin-1. Chinese J Integrative Medicine. 2009,29(1):60-64.

She Weimin, Hu Dechang, Zhou Zhaohui, Gu Weiguang and Wang Jiyao. Clinical study of Ganping Capsule to treat fibrotic patients with chronic hepatitis B. Chinese Hepatol. 2002,7(4):254-255.

Xu Lieming, Liu Ping, Liu Cheng, Gu Hongtu, Xue Huiming, Lv Gang and Li Fenghua. Action of Fuzheng Huayu 319 decoction on liver fibrosis in chronic hepatitis B Chinese J Hepatol. 1997,5(4):207-209.

Xu Lieming, Liu Cheng and Liu Ping. Effect of lithospermate B on proliferation and shape of rat hepatic Fat-storing cells and production of extracellular matrix *in vitro*. Chinese J Hepatol. 1996,4(2):86-89.

Liu Ping, Zhu Dayuan, Hu Yiyang, Jiang Fuxiang, Liu Cheng, Wang Baode, Xu Lieming, Jiang Shanhao, Liu Chenghai and Zhang Zhiqing. Study of Salvianolic-acid B on anti-fibrosis in chronic hepatitis B. Bulletin of Medical Research 2003,32(2):16-17.

L Xu, A Y Hui, E Albanis, M J Arthur, S M O'Byrne, WS Blaner, P Mukherjee, S L Friedman, F J Eng. Human Hepatic Stellate Cell Lines, LX-1 and LX-2: New Tools for Analysis of Hepatic Fibrosis. *Gut* 2005;54:142-151.

7

Role of Manganese as Mediator of Central Nervous System: Alteration in Experimental Portal Hypertension

Juan Pablo Prestifilippo[1,2], Silvina Tallis[2], Amalia Delfante[2], Pablo Souto[2], Juan Carlos Perazzo[2] and Gabriela Beatriz Acosta[1,2]

[1]*Institute of Pharmacological Research (ININFA), National Research Council of Argentina (CONICET) and Department of Pathophysiology, School of Pharmacy and Biochemistry, University of Buenos Aires, Buenos Aires,*

[2]*Laboratory of Portal Hypertension, School of Pharmacy and Biochemistry & Hepatic Encephalopathy, University of Buenos Aires, Buenos Aires, Argentina*

1. Introduction

Portal hypertension (PH) is a major syndrome that frequently accompany chronic liver diseases such as cirrhosis. Prehepatic PH develops a splanchnic hyperdynamic circulation and hyperemia with increased splanchnic resistance and production of collateral vessels that drive splanchnic blood flow to systemic circulation (Chojkier & Groszmann, 1981). Several substances have been proposed as mediators of this hypodynamic circulatory state including prostacyclins, nitric oxide and endotoxins (Bosch et al., 1992; Reiner & Groszmann, 1999; Palma et al., 2005). PH is found in patients with cirrhosis, and in portal vein thrombosis. It is characterized by an increase in splanchnic blood flow and pressure, among others caused by abdominal blood flow resistance, secondary to important liver parenchyma alterations (fibrosis or cirrhosis).

Recent studies have demonstrated that experimental PH in rats is also a sub-clinic model of Minimal Hepatic Encephalopathy (MHE) (Butterworth et al., 2009), since rats with PH develop hyperammonemia, electrophysiology alterations, blood-brain barrier (BBB) breakdown, hippocampal mitochondrial dysfunction and changes in frontal cortex and hippocamus on glutamate uptake (Scorticati et al., 2004; Lores-Arnaiz et al., 2005; Eizayaga et al., 2006; Acosta et al., 2009; Bustamante et al., 2011).

Chronic hepatic encephalopathy (HE) is a complex neuropsychiatric syndrome associated with liver dysfunction, such as cirrhosis. The pathophysiology of HE is poorly understood and there are few high-quality diagnostic tests and markers. As a result, its treatment has improved only slightly over the last several decades (Zafirova & O'Connor, 2010). The current classificaton of HE is: Type A HE associated with acute liver failure, Type B with portosystemic bypass without intrinsic liver disease and Type C with cirrhosis (Merino et al., 2011; Ferenci et al., 2002). In chronic liver dysfunction, such as cirrhosis, it occurs more insidiously causing a range of neuropsychiatric disturbances which include psychomotor dysfunction, impaired memory, increased reaction time, sensory abnormalities and poor concentration (Albrecht, 1998; Scorticati et al., 2005; Albrecht et al., 2007). In its severest forms, patients may develop confusion, stupor, coma and death (Ferenci et al., 2002).

Hyperammonemia is a well-known toxic substance for the central nervous system (CNS), especially when levels exceed the antitoxic capacity of the brain cells. Arterial blood ammonia concentrations are frequently elevated in patients with portal-systemic encephalopathy and studies in experimental animal models of chronic liver failure reveal blood and brain ammonia concentrations approaching the millimolar range (normal range 0.05-0.10 mM) (Butterworth, 1991; Therrien et al., 1991).

The CNS is an important target for manganese (Mn), an essential element that is normally excreted via the hepatobiliary route (Papavasiliou et al., 1966; Teeguarden et. al., 2007). Manganese has a key role in the normal functioning of several enzymes including mitochondrial superoxide dismutase, glutamine synthetase, and phosphoenolpyruvate carboxykinase (Bentle et al., 1976; Stallings et al., 1991). The metal was first considered to be neurotoxic more than 150 years ago, when workers employed in grinding black oxide of Mn developed an unsteady gait and muscle weakness (Couper, 1837). Since that time, many cases of Mn neurotoxicity (manganism), a neurologic disease characterized by psychological and neurologic abnormalities, have been reported, particularly in miners, smelters, welders, and workers involved in the alloy industry (Mena et al., 1967; Eamara et al., 1971).

As manganese acts as a cofactor for many enzymes and therefore, it plays important biological functions (Keen et al., 1984). Nevertheless, high concentration of Mn exerts toxic effects in the brain (Yamada et al., 1986) and the accumulation of Mn in the basal ganglia produces an irreversible neurological syndrome similar to Parkinson's disease. Typically, patients exhibit extrapyramidal changes that include hypokinesia, rigidity and tremor (Cotzias, 1958; Mena, 1974). High levels of this metal can cause alterations in development as well as reproductive dysfunction (Grey & Laskey, 1980; Laskey et al., 1982). Manganese deficiencies produce impairment of growth and reproduction in rats of both sexes (Boyer et al., 1942; Smith et al., 1944; Prestifilippo et al., 2008). Manganese exists as divalent and trivalent forms in the plasma (Nandedkav et al., 1973; Scheuhammer and Cherian, 1985) and both may be transported into the brain across the BBB and reach the blood–cerebral spinal fluid (CSF) and accumulates in the brain (Aschner 1992; 1999).

Importantly, these not only occurs in animal models but in human since the patients with chronic liver failure have been shown to exhibit increased serum and brain levels of Mn and display many of the clinical and pathological features associated with manganese toxicity (Krieger et al., 1995; Spahr et al., 1996; Hauser et al., 1994; 1996; Sassine et al., 2002). Excessive deposition of Mn in brain has also been demonstrated in a rat model of cirrhosis (Rose et al., 1999). This elevation is believed to be due to decrease elimination of manganese via biliary excretion (Papavasiliou et al., 1966; Teeguarden et al., 2007), and to increase systemic availability due to portal-systemic shunting associated with chronic liver disease (Spahr et al., 1996; Rose et al., 1999).

1.1 Study of the effect of manganese in plasma and hypothalamus levels in portal hypertensive rats

Different studies indicated that participation of manganese in HE (Hauser et al., 1994; Matsuda et al., 1994; Krieger et al., 1995; Pomier-Layrargues et al., 1995; Siger-Zajde et al., 2002). Therefore we determinate manganese concentration on plasma and the effects of this metal in hypothalamus in PH rats.

1.2 Investigate the action of manganese of manganese on amino acids and nitric oxide levels

Amino acids play an important role in the maintenance of homeostasis on the brain. Considering that manganese may also have a role in the pathogenesis of chronic HE (Hauser et al., 1994; Matsuda et al., 1994; Krieger et al., 1995; Poimier-Layrargues et al., 1995). The second point was to analyze the effects of manganese on amino acids levels in hypothalamus using the same animal model.

The third point to consider in this work was whether changes produced by manganese in PH may be due to the mechanism of nitric oxide pathway.

2. Materials and methods

2.1 Animals and surgical procedures

Adult male Wistar rats (240–260 g of body weight) were kept under controlled conditions of light (12 h light/dark cycle: 8 a.m. to 8 p.m.). They were housed under constant temperature and a 12-hour light-dark cycle and kept in an acclimatized animal room (21-23 °C) with *ad libitum* access to dry food and tap water. Special care for perfect air renewal was taken.

All animal procedures were performed in accordance with our institutional guidelines after obtaining the permission of the Laboratory Animal Committee and with the U.S. National Institute of Health Guide for the Care and Use of Laboratory Animals (NIH publication N*8* 80-23/96).

Prehepatic PH in rats was induced by a calibrated stenosis of the portal vein according to Chojkier & Groszmann (1981). Rats were lightly anesthetized with ether and then a midline abdominal incision was made. The portal vein was located and isolated from surrounding tissues. A ligature of 3.0 silk sutures was placed around the vein, and snugly tied to a 20-gauge blunt-end needle placed alongside the portal vein. The needle was subsequently removed to yield a calibrated stenosis of the portal vein, after which the abdominal incision was sutured. Operations were performed at 2 p.m. to obey circadian rhythm. Fourteen days after portal vein ligation, animals exhibit an increase in portal pressure. Sham-operated rats underwent the same experimental procedure, except that the portal vein was isolated but not stenosed. Animals were placed in individual cages and allowed to recover from surgery. Rats were sacrificed by decapitation at two weeks after surgery.

All efforts were made to minimize suffering of animals and to reduce the number of animals used.

2.2 Portal pressure measurement

Fourteen days after the corresponding operation, the rats were anesthetized with intraperitoneal sodium pentobarbital (40 mg/kg). Portal pressure was measured through a needle placed in the splenic pulp, and maintained in place by cyanoacrylate gel. The needle was cannulated to a polyethylene catheter (50) filled with a heparinized saline solution (25 U/mL), and connected to a Statham Gould P23ID pressure transducer (Statham, Hato Rey, Puerto Rico), coupled to a Grass 79D polygraph (Grass Instruments, Quincy, MA, USA).

2.3 Determination of plasma ammonia

Blood samples were obtained by abdominal aortic artery puncture for the determination of biochemical parameters. Ammoniac Enzymatic UV kits (Biomerieux-France) were used to determine plasma ammonia concentration.

	Sham operated	**PH**
Portal pressure (mmHg)	7.3±1.4	13.5±1.3*
Plasma Ammonia(µm/L)	26±4	82±17 **

Table 1. Determination of portal pressure and plasma ammonia levels

Portal pressure was 7.3 ± 1.4 mm Hg in the sham-operated group versus PH group vs 13.5 ± 1.3 mm Hg by an enhanced 184% (* $p<0.05$). In other hand, plasma ammonium levels was 26 ± 4 µm/L in the sham-operated group versus PH group was 82 ± 17 µm/L, by an increase of 315% (** $p<0.01$).

2.4 Determination of manganese levels and in Hypothalamus

For the determination of manganese levels in tissue, brains were rapidly dissected and the hypothalamus was removed. Tissue blocks were snap frozen in liquid nitrogen and saved at -80 °C and blood was digested by digestion in oxidizing acid, both were analysis by inductively coupled plasma mass spectrometry as described (Melnyk et al., 2003). The method was considered in Sham operated when the duplicates were ± 15% of the expected value and blank values were < 0.001 ppb.

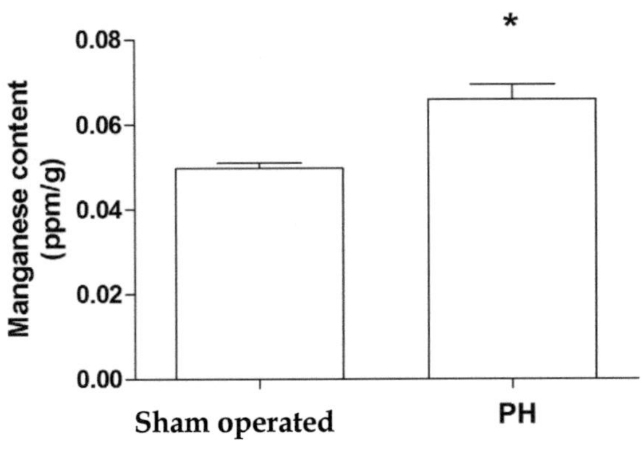

Fig. 1. Manganese analyses. A significant increase of manganese (*$p < 0.05$) was observed in plasma levels in PH groups compared with the respective Sham operated.

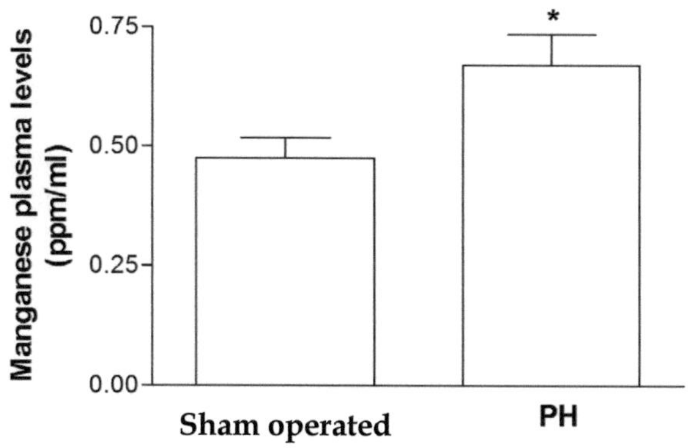

Fig. 2. Effects of Manganese on hypothalamus. The stenosis of the portal vein produced an accumulation of Manganese in the brain by 14 days after surgery versus sham operated resulting an increase in Manganese levels in hypothalamus *($p < 0.05$).

2.5 In vivo studies

The rats were anesthetized (ketamian/xilasiana) and implanted a cannula into the lateral cerebral ventricle, using a stereotaxic instrument and coordinates from the atlas. The correct localization of the cannula in the ventricle was confirmed at the end of the experiment. The experiments were performed a week after the implantation of the cannula. The day of experiment, conscious, freely moving rats were divided into two groups of 10 animals each. The rats were microinjected intracerebroventricularly (i.c.v.) during 1 min with 5 µl of sterile saline (control group) or 10 µg of MnCl2/5 µl sterile saline. After decapitation, the brains were rapidly dissected and the hypothalamus was removed. All incubations were carried out in a Dubnoff shaker (50 cycles per min; 95% O_2/5% CO_2) at 37°C. The hypothalami (seven to eight for each group) were preincubated individually in glass tubes in 500µl of Krebs-Ringer bicarbonate-buffered medium (NaCl 124.40 mM, KCl 4.98 mM, NaHCO3 24.88 mM, CaCl2 1.50 mM, MgCl2 1.42 mM, KH2PO4 1.25mM containing 0.1% glucose, pH: 7.4). After this preincubation (15 min) the medium was discarded and replaced with fresh medium alone or containing the substances to be tested. The incubation continued for 30 min. At the end of the incubation period the media were removed and the tissues were homogenized and submitted to appropriate extraction procedure and stored at −20 °C until the respective assays were conducted.

2.6 NOS enzimatic activity determination

Determination of NOS activity was performed by a modification (Canteros et al., 1995) of the ^{14}C-arginine method of Bredt & Snyder (1989). After the incubation period (30 min) the hypothalamus were immediately homogenized in 0.5 ml of N-(2-hydroxyethyl)-piperazine-N-2-ethanesulfonic acid (HEPES) (20mM, pH: 7.4) with addition of $CaCl_2$ (1.25mM) and DL-dithiothreitol (DTT, 1mM). The reaction was started by adding NADPH (nicotinamide adenine dinucleotide phosphate, reduced) (120µM) and 200.000 dpm of ^{14}C-arginine (360 mCi/mmol) to the homogenates. The tubes were incubated for 15 min at

37°C in a Dubnoff metabolic shaker (50 cycles per min and 95%O_2;5%CO_2 atmosphere). At the end of this incubation period, the tubes were immediately centrifuged at 10.000 g for 10 min at 4°C. The supernatants were immediately applied to individual columns containing 1 ml of Dowex AG 50 W-X8 200 mesh sodium form, and washed with 2.0 ml of double distilled water. All collected fluid from each column was counted for ^{14}C-citrulline activity in a scintillation counter. NOS converts arginine into equimolar quantities of citrulline and NO, the data were expressed as pmol of NO produced per hypothalamus per min.

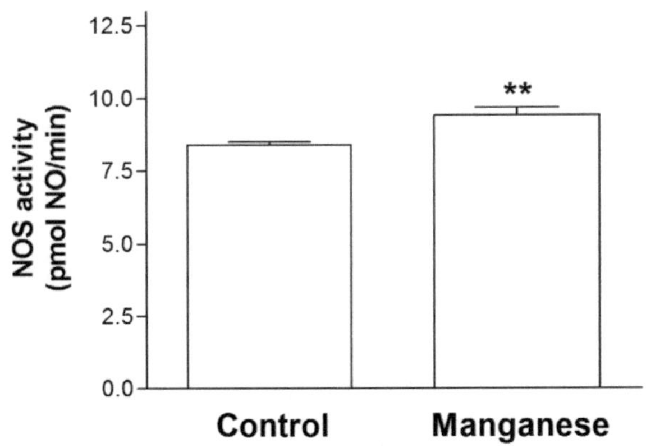

Fig. 3. Determination of NOS activity. Results show that Manganese increased NOS activity (**$p<0.01$) evaluated by the conversion of ^{14}C-arginine into ^{14}C-citrulline compared with the control group.

2.7 Quantification of GABA, aspartate and glutamate

The method described by Durkin et al. (1988) allowed the isolation of γ-aminobutiric acid (GABA), aspartate and glutamate. Aliquots of 50 µl of homogenates were mixed with 400 µl of O-phthalaldehyde, 50 µl of 2-mercaptoethanol in 50 µl of ethanol, and 400 µl of 0.5 M sodium borate, pH 9 (reaction mixture). After 30 min at room temperature, 50 µl of the reaction mixture were injected into the HPLC column. The O-phthalaldehyde derivates were then separated on a reverse-phase column and eluted with a buffer of acetonitrile/sodium acetate 1:9 (v/v), pH 4 at a flow rate of 1.6 ml/min. The concentrations of amino acids were extrapolated from curves made with known amounts of standard amino acids.

Different functions of the CNS are mediated by the action of diverse amino acids neurotransmitters such as aspartate, glutamate and GABA. Therefore, with the purpose of determining whether manganese could affect their secretions, evaluating the release and the content of aspartate, glutamate and GABA from the hypothalamus obtained after i.c.v. injection of manganese determined by high-performance liquid chromatography (HPLC). GABA release by 2 folds (* $p< 0.05$) compared with the respective control group. The others neurotransmitters not shown significative differences.

	Aspartate		Glutamate		GABA	
	Release	Content	Release	Content	Release	Content
Control	192 ± 11	1505± 171	157±10	309± 39	78 ± 7	84 ± 24
Manganese	206± 11	1679± 63	163± 9	271± 47	106± 7 *	115 ±21

Table 2. Release and concentration of different amino acids such as aspartate, glutamate and GABA following the injection of manganese.

2.8 Drugs, chemicals and radiolabeled compounds

Manganese chloride (MnCl2) was purchased from Anedra (San Fernando, Buenos Aires, Argentina). HEPES, DTT, NADPH, Glutamate, Aspartate and GABA were purchased from Sigma Aldrich (St Louis, MO , USA). Dowex AG 50 W-X8 200-400 mesh sodium form was obtained from Bio-Rad (Hercules, CA), and the ^{14}C-arginine-monohydrochloride 360 mCi/mmol was from Amersham Pharmacia (Buckinghamshire, HP, UK). All other chemical materials used in this work were from analytical grade.

2.9 Statistical analysis

Experiments were repeated at least twice employing seven to eight animals per group in each experiment. All data are expressed as the mean ± SEM. Comparisons between groups were performed by using a one-way ANOVA followed by the Student-Newman-Keuls multiple comparison tests for unequal replicates. Student's t-test was used when comparing two groups. Differences with p values < 0.05 were considered significant.

3. Conclusions

Experimental prehepatic PH produces a hyperdynamic redistribution of splanchnic circulation and minimal liver damage. Ammonia was considerate the major responsible of the alterations in CNS included cytotoxic brain edema characterized by swelling of astrocyte. However the ammonia is not the only toxic and as Shawcross & Jalan (2005) demonstrated the participation of other relevant metabolic molecules such as manganese.

In the present work we showed for the first time that rats with experimental prehepatic PH presented increase of manganese level in plasma and hyphotalamus. The manganese is transported to the liver after absorption from the gut and the liver may be important as a deposit for manganese, with hepatic manganese later delivered to the brain (Takeda, 1998). Rats with PH show a redistribution of splanchnic circulation and increase the different toxic in blood including ammonia and manganese as shown in this work. Even more, patients with abnormal deposit of manganese in the basal ganglia has been estimated by magnetic resonance imaging was associated with the elevated levels of manganese in the blood (Krieger et al., 1995; Siger-Zajdel et al., 2002).

This metal is able to enter the brain through the cerebral vasculature and the spinal fluid. The mechanism by which Mn crosses the BBB is not yet well understood, but involves binding of the metal to transport systems such as transferrin (Aschner & Aschner, 1992; 1999). Also, as Mn levels rise in blood, the influx into the spinal fluid rises and entry across the choroid plexus becomes more important (Murphy et al., 1991). Importantly, Mn accumulates in the hypothalamus (Deskin et al., 1980; Pine et al., 2005) and is known to be taken up by both neurons and glial cells (Tholey et al., 1990) and, hence, suggesting a potential role in neuronal/glial communications within the developing hypothalamus.

We investigated the participation of hypothalamus NO production and we found that the rats with administer this metal increased the activity of NOS. So we can deduce that nitric oxide has been involved in this pathophysiological brain processes

This metal is able to enter the brain through the cerebral vasculature and the spinal fluid. The mechanism by which manganese crosses the BBB is not yet well understood, but involves binding of the metal to transport systems such as transferrin (Aschner & Aschner, 1992; 1999). On the other hand, has been observed a decrease of GABA concentration opposite to the chronic exhibition to manganese in certain regions of the CNS as the globo pallidum, but not in substance nigra or hippocampus (Bonilla et al., 1994; Zwingmann et al., 2003). This effect on GABA levels produces to itself across the direct action of the manganese on the expression of glutamic decarboxylase, enzyme that regulates GABA synthesis (Tomas-Camardiel et al., 2002).

When the Mn is accumulated in the synapsis it produces a consistent neuropathy with an excitocitotoxic effect, suggesting that the mechanism of glutamate is involved in the development of the pathology described by the manganese. These findings suggest that the manganese induce an increase in nitric oxide synthase production probably correlated to GABAergic and glutamatergic hypothalamic neurons that form a part of a network neuronal autoregulation.

4. Acknowledgment

This work was supported in part by grants UBACYT ; B019 and B101 from the University of Buenos Aires and PIP N° 114-2009-0100118 from National Scientific and Technologic Research Council (CONICET) to GBA. GBA is member of CONICET.

5. References

Acosta G.B.; Fernández M.A.; Roselló D.M.; Tomaro M.L.; Balestrasse K. & Lemberg A. (2009). Glutamine synthetase activity and glutamate uptake in hippocampus and frontal cortex in portal hypertensive rats. World J Gastroenterol, Vol. 21, N° 15, pp. 2893-2899.

Albrecht, J. (1998) Roles of neuroactive amino acids in ammonia neurotoxicity. J Neurosci Res Vol., 51, pp. 133-138.

Albrecht, J.; Sonnewald, U.; Waagepetersen, H.S. & Schousboe, A. (2007). Glutamine in the central nervous system: function and dysfunction. Front Biosci Vol. 12, pp. 332-343.

Aschner, M.; Gannon, M. & Kimelberg, H.K. (1992). Manganese uptake and efflux in cultured rat astrocytes. J Neurochem Vol. 58, pp. 730–735.

Aschner, M.; Vrana, K.E. & Zheng, W. (1999). Manganese uptake and distribution in the central nervous system (CNS). Neurotoxicology, Vol. 20, pp. 173–180.

Bentle, L.A. & Lardy, H.A. (1976). Interaction of anions and divalent metal ions with phosphoenolpyruvate carboxykinase. J Biol Chem. Vol. 251, pp. 2916–2921.

Bonilla, E.; Arrieta, A.; Castro, F.; Dávila, J.O. & Quiroz, I. (1994). Manganese toxicity: free amino acids in the striatum and olfactory bulb of the mouse. Invest Clin. Vol. 35, N°4, pp. 175-81.

Bosch, J.; Pizcueta, P.; Feu, F.; Fernández, M. & Garcia-Pagan, J.C. (1992). Pathophysiology of portal hypertension. Gastroenterol Clin North Am, Vol. 21, pp. 1–14.

Boyer, P.H.; Shaw, J.H. & Phillips, P.H. (1942). Studies on manganese deficiency in the rat. J. Biol. Chem. Vol. 143, pp. 417-425.

Bredt, D.S. & Snyder, S.H. (1989) Nitric oxide mediates glutamate-linked enhancement of cGMP levels in the cerebellum. Proc. Natl. Acad. Sci. U. S. A. Vol. 86, pp. 9030-9033.

Bustamante, J.; Lorez-Arnaiz, S.; Tallis, S.; Roselló, D.M.; Lago, N.; Lemberg, A.; Boveris, A. & Perazzo, J.C. (2011). Mitochondrial dysfunction as a mediator of hippocampal apoptosis in a model of hepatic encephalopathy. Mol Cell Biochem. Vol. 354, N° (1-2), pp. 231-240

Butterworth, R.F. (1991). Pathophysiology of hepatic encephalopathy: the ammonia hypothesis revisited. In (F. Bengtsson, ed.) Progress in Hepatic Encephalopathy and Metabolic Nitrogen Exchange, CRC Press, Boca Raton, pp. 9-24.

Butterworth, R.F. (2000). Complications of cirrhosis III. Hepatic encephalopathy. J Hepatol Vol. 32, pp. 171–180.

Butterworth, R.F.; Norenberg, M.D.; Felipo, V.; Ferenci, P.; Albrecht, J.; Blei. A.T. & Members of the ISHEN Commission on Experimental Models of HE. (2009). Experimental models of hepatic encephalopathy: ISHEN guidelines. Liver Int. Vol. 29, N° 6, pp. 783-788.

Canteros, G.; Rettori, V.; Franchi, A.; Genaro, A.M.; Cebral, E.; Faletti, A.; Gimeno, M. & McCann, S.M. (1995). Ethanol inhibits luteinizing hormone-releasing hormone (LHRH) secretion by blocking the response of LHRH neuronal terminals to nitric oxide. Proc. Natl. Acad. Sci. U. S. A. Vol. 92, pp. 3416-3420.

Chojkier, M. & Groszmann, R.J. (1981) Measurement of portal-systemic shunting in the rat by using gamma-label microspheres. Am J Physiol Vol. 240, G 371-375.

Cotzias, G.C. (1958). Manganese in health and disease. Physiol. Rev. Vol. 38, pp. 503-553.

Couper, J. (1837). On the effects of black oxide of manganese when inhaled into the lungs. Br Ann Med Pharmacol Vol. 1, pp. 41–42.

Deskin, R.; Bursain, S.J.& Edens, F.W. (1980). Neurochemical alterations induced by manganese chloride in neonatal rats. Neurotoxicology Vol. 2, pp. 65-73.

Durkin, T.A.; Anderson, G.M. & Cohen. D.J. (1988). HPLC analysis of neurotransmitter amino acids in brain. J. Chromatogr. Vol. 428, pp. 9–15.

Eizayaga, F.; Scorticati, C.; Prestifilippo, J.P.; Romay, S.; Fernández, M.A.; Castro J.L.; Lemberg, A. & Perazzo, J.C. (2006). Altered blood-brain barrier permeability in rats with prehepatic portal hypertension turns to normal when portal pressure is lowered. World J Gastroenterol Vol. 12, pp. 1367–1372.

Emara, A.M.; el-Ghawabi, S.H.; Madkour, O.I. & el-Samra, G.H.(1971). Chronic manganese poisoning in the dry battery industry. Br J Ind Med Vol. 28, Vol. 1, pp. 78–82.

Ferenci, P.; Lockwood, A.; Muller, K.; Tarter, R.; Weissenborn, K. & Blei, A.T. (2002). Hepatic encephalopathy-definition, nomenclature, diagnosis and quantification. Final report of the working party at the 11th World Congress of Gastroenterology, Vienna 1998. Hepatology Vol. 35, pp. 716–721.

Giordano, G.; Pizzurro, D.; Vandemark, K.; Guizzetti, M. & Costa, L.G. (2009). Manganese inhibits the ability of astrocytes to promote neuronal differentiation. Toxicol Appl Pharmacol. Vol. 240, N°2, pp. 226-35.

Glowinski, J. & Iversen, L.L. (1966). Regional studies of catecholamines in the rat brain. I. The disposition of [^{3}H]norepinephrine, [^{3}H]dopamine and [^{3}H]dopa in various regions of the brain. J Neurochem Vol. 13, pp. 655-669.

Grey, L.E. & Laskey, J.W. (1980). Multivariate analysis of the effects of manganese on the reproductive physiology and behavior of the male house mouse. J. Toxicol. Environ. Health. Vol. 6, pp. 861-867.

Hauser, R.; Zesiewicz, T.A.; Rosemurgy, A.S.; Martinez,C. & Olanow, C.W. (1994). Manganese intoxication and chronic liver failure. Ann. Neurol. Vol. 36, pp. 871-875.

Hauser, R.A.; Zesiewicz, T. A.; Martinez, C.; Rosemurgy, A.S. & Olanow, C. W. (1996). Blood manganese correlates with brain magnetic resonance imaging changes in patients with liver disease. Can. J. Neurol. Sci. Vol. 23, pp 95–98.

Keen, C.L.; Lonnerdal, B. & Hurley, L.S. (1984). Manganese. In: Biochemistry of the essential ultratrace elements. E. Frieden, (Ed.) pp. 89-132, New York: Plenum Press.

Krieger D.; Krieger, S.; Jansen, O.; Gass, P.; Theilmann, L. & Lichtnecker, H. (1995). Manganese and chronic hepatic encephalopathy. Lancet Vol. 346, pp. 270–274.

Laskey, J.W.; Rehnberg, J.F. & Hein, J.F. (1982). Effects of chronic manganese exposure on selected reproductive parameters. J. Toxicol. Environ. Health. Vol. 9, pp. 677-687.

Lores-Arnaiz, S.; Perazzo, J.C.; Prestifilippo, J.P.; Lago, N.; D'Amico, G.; Czerniczyniec, A.; Bustamante, J.; Boveris, A. & Lemberg, A. (2005). Hippocampal mitochondrial dysfunction with decreased mtNOS activity in prehepatic portal hypertensive rats. Neurochem Int. Vol. 47, pp. 362–368.

Matsuda, A.; Kimura, M.; Takeda, T.; Kataoka, M.; Sato, M. & Itokawa, Y. (1994) . Changes in manganese content of mononuclear blood cells in patients receiving total parenteral nutrition. Clin. Chem. Vol. 40, pp. 829–832.

McCarty, J. H. (2005). Cell biology of the neurovascular unit: implications for drug delivery across the blood-brain barrier. Assay Drug Dev. Technol. Vol. 3, N°1, pp. 89–95.

Melnyk, L.J.; Morgan, J.N.; Fernando, R.; Pellizzari, E.D. & Akinbo, O. (2003). Determination of metals in composite diet samples by inductively coupled plasma-mass spectrometry. J. AOAC Int. Vol. 86, pp. 439- 447.

Mena, I. (1974). The role of manganese in human disease. Ann. Clin. Chem. Vol. 214, pp. 489-495

Mena, I.; Marin, O.; Fuenzalida, S. & Cotzias, G.C. (1967). Chronic manganese poisoning: clinical picture and manganese turnover. Neurology Vol. 17, N° 2, pp.128–136.

Merino, J.; Aller, M.A.; Rubio, S.; Arias, N.; Nava, M.P.; Loscertales, M.; Arias, J. & Arias, J.L. (2011) Gut-brain chemokine changes in portal hypertensive rats. Dig. Dis. Sci. Vol. 56; N° 8, pp. 2309-2317.

Murphy, V.A.; Wadhawami, K.C.; Smith, O.R. & Rapoport, S.I. (1991). Saturable transport of manganese across the rat blood brain barrier. J. Neurochem. Vol. 57, pp. 948-954.

Nandedkar, A.K.; Nurse, C.E.& Friedberg, F. (1973) Mn++ binding by plasma proteins. Int J Pept Protein Res. Vol. 5, N°4, pp. 279-281.

Nandedkar, A.K.N.; Nurse, C.E. & Friedberg, F. (1973). Mn binding by plasma proteins, Int. J. Pept. Protein Res. Vol. 5, pp. 279–281.

Pal, K.P.; Samii, A. & Clane, D.B. (1999). Manganese neurotoxicity: A review of clinical features, imaging and pathology. Neurotoxicology Vol. 20, pp. 227-238.

Palma, M.D.; Aller, M.A.; Vara, E.; Nava, M.P.; García, C.; Arias-Diaz. J.; Balibrea, J.L. & Arias, J. (2005). Portal hypertension produces an evolutive hepato-intestinal pro- and anti-inflammatory response in the rat. Cytokine Vol. 31, pp. 213- 226.

Papavasiliou, P.S.; Miller, S.T.; & Cotzias, G.C. (1966). Role of liver in regulating distribution and excretion of manganese. Am J Physiol Vol. 211, N° 1, pp. 211-216.

Pomier-Layrargues, G.; Spahr, L.; & Butterworth, R.F. (1995). Increased manganese concentrations in pallidum of cirrhotic patients. Lancet Vol. 345, N° 8951, pp. 735.

Prestifilippo, J.P.; Fernández-Solari, J.; De Laurentiis, A.; Mohn, C.E.; de la Cal C.; Reynoso, R.; Dees, W.L. & Rettori, V. (2008). Acute effect of manganese on hypothalamic luteinizing hormone releasing hormone secretion in adult male rats: involvement of specific neurotransmitter systems. Toxicol Sci. Vol. 105, N°2, pp. 295-302.

Rama Rao, K.V.; Reddy, P.V.; Hazell, A.S. & Norenberg, M.D. (2007). Manganese induces cell swelling in cultured astrocytes. Neurotoxicology Vol.28, N°4, pp. 807-812.

Reiner, W. & Groszmann, R. (1999). Nitric oxide and portal hypertension: its role in the regulation of intrahepatic and splanchnic vascular resistance. Semin Liver Dis Vol. 19, pp. 411-426.

Rose, C.; Butterworth, R. F.; Zayed, J.; Normandin, L.; Todd, K.; Michalak, A.; Sphar, L.; Huet, P.M. & Pomier- Layrargues, G. (1999). Manganese deposition in basal ganglia structures results from both portal-systemic shunting and liver dysfunction. Gastroenterology Vol. 117, N°3, pp. 640-644.

Sassine, M. P.; Mergler, D.; Bowler, R. & Hudnell, H.K.(2002). Manganese accentuates adverse mental health effects associated with alcohol use disorders. Biol. Psychiatry Vol. 51, pp. 909-921.

Scheuhammer, A.M. &, Cherian, M.G. (1985). Binding of manganese in human and rat plasma. Biochim Biophys Acta Vol. 840, N°2, pp. 163-169.

Scorticati, C.; Prestifilippo, J.P.; Eizayaga, F.X.; Castro. J.L.; Romay, S.; Fernández, M.A.; Lemberg, A. & Perazzo, J.C. (2004). Hyperammonemia, brain edema and blood-brain barrier alterations in prehepatic portal hypertensive rats and paracetamol intoxication. World J Gastroenterol Vol. 10, pp. 1321-1324.

Shawcross, D. & Jalan, R. (2005). The pathophysiologic basis of hepatic encephalopathy: central role for ammonia and inflammation. Cell Mol Life Sci., Vol. 62, N°19-20, pp. 2295-2304.

Siger-Zajdel, M. & Selmaj, K. (2002). Hyperintense basal ganglia on T1-weighted magnetic resonance images in a patient with common variable immunodeficiency associated with elevated serum manganese. J. Neuroimag. Vol.12, pp. 84-86.

Smith, S.E.; Medlicott, M. & Ellis, G.H. (1944). Manganese deficiency in the rabbit. Arch. Biochem. Biophys. Vol. 4, pp 81-289.

Spahr, L.; Butterworth, R. F.; Fontaine, S.; Bui, L.; Therrien, G.; Milette, P. C.; Lebrun, L. H.; Zayed, J.; Leblanc, A. & Pomier-Layrargues, G. (1996). Increased blood manganese in cirrhotic patients: Relationship to pallidal magnetic resonance signal hyperintensity and neurological symptoms. Hepatology Vol. 24, pp.1116-1120.

Stallings, W.C.; Metzger, A.L.; Pattridge, K.A.; Fee, J.A. & Ludwig ML (1991) Structure-function relationships in iron and manganese superoxide dismutases. Free Radic Res Commu. Vol. 12-13, N° 1, pp. 259-268

Takeda, A.; Sawashita, J. & Okada, S. (1998). Manganese concentration in rat brain: manganese transport from the peripheral tissues. Neurosci. Lett. Vol. 242, pp. 45–48.

Teeguarden, J.G.; Dorman, D.C.; Nong, A.; Covington, T.R.; Clewell, H.J, 3rd. & Andersen, M.E. (2007). Pharmacokinetic modeling of manganese. II. Hepatic processing after ingestion and inhalation. J Toxicol Environ Health A. Vol. 70, N° 18, pp.1505-1514.

Therrien, G; Giguère, J.F. & Butterworth, R.F. (1991). Increased cerebrospinal fluid lactate reflects deterioration of neurological status in experimental portal-systemic encephalopathy. Metab Brain Dis. Vol. 6, N°4, pp. 225-231.

Tholey, G.; Megias-Megias, L.; Wedler, F.C. & Ledig, M. (1990). Modulation of Mn accumulation in cultured rat neuronal and astroglial cells. Neurochem. Res. Vol.15, pp. 751-754.

Tomás-Camardiel, M.; Herrera, A.J.; Venero, J.L.; Cruz Sánchez-Hidalgo, M.; Cano, J. & Machado, A. (2002). Differential regulation of glutamic acid decarboxylase mRNA and tyrosine hydroxylase mRNA expression in the aged manganese-treated rats. Brain Res Mol Brain Res. Vol. 103, N° 1-2, pp. 116-129.

Uchida, S.; Kitamoto, A.; Umeeda, H.; Nakagawa, N.; Masushige, S. & Kida, S. (2005) Chronic reduction in dietary tryptophan leads to changes in the emotional response to stress in mice. J Nutr Sci Vitaminol Vol. 51, pp. 175-181.

Yamada, M.; Ohno, S.; Okayasu, I.; Hatakeyama, S.; Watanabe, H. ; Ushio, K. & Tsukagoshi, H. (1986). Chronic manganese poisoning: A neuropathological study with determination of manganese distribution in the brain. Acta Neuropathol. Vol. 70, pp. 273-278.

Zafirova, Z. & O'Connor, M. (2010). Hepatic encephalopathy: current management strategies and treatment, including management and monitoring of cerebral edema and intracraneal hypertension in fulminant hepatic failure. Current Opinion Anaesthesiol. Vol. 23, pp. 121– 127.

8

Changes of Peripheral Blood Cells in Patients with Cirrhotic Portal Hypertension

Lv Yunfu
People's Hospital of Hainan Province,
Haikou, Hainan Province,
China

1. Introduction

Hemocytopenia is very common in patients with cirrhotic portal hypertension. These patients experience complications of monolineage or multi-lineage peripheral cytopenias. However, the range of variation of these cytopenias is unclear, and the question of whether they affect all patients remains uncertain. In general, it is believed that such cytopenias are caused by hypersplenism; however, this may not always be the case as numerous factors that cause hemocytopenia exist, and hypersplenism is only one of them. Patients with hypersplenism experience hemocytopenia, but not all cytopenias are caused by hypersplenism.

Can cytopenias be graded? How do cytopenias affect prognosis? According to the observation of clinical cases, cytopenias may, in fact, influence prognosis. These questions will be discussed in this chapter, which integrates clinical data from 366 cases investigated by the author.

2. Changes of peripheral blood cells

It has been accepted that "all patients with splenomegaly due to cirrhotic portal hypertension will manifest cytopenias in peripheral blood [1]; however, certain limitations were noticed in the traditional opinion by the author after studying clinical data from 366 cases.

This study included 250 male patients and 116 female patients (a total of 366 patients), and the ratio of males to females was 2.2:1. The patients' ages ranged from 5 to 79 years, with an average of 43 years. All the patients had hepatic cirrhosis and an enlarged spleen. The average spleen size was 224mm×159mm×95mm, as measured by B ultrasound or CT scan. Upper gastrointestinal imaging and gastroscopy revealed that there were medium-to-severe varices in the distal esophagus and gastric fundus (Figure 1). Seventy-four patients (20.2%) were hospitalized for gastrointestinal hemorrhage, and 248 (67.8%) patients had previously experienced hemorrhaging.Thirty-six patients (9.8%) had a normal blood cell count and 330 patients had peripheral cytopenias, in which mono-lineage cytopenias accounted for 30% (99/330), bi-lineage cytopenias accounted for 35.8% (118/330) and tri-lineage cytopenias accounted for 34.2% (113/330).The range of variation of hemocytopenia is listed in Table 1. Two-hundred ninety-seven cases underwent bone marrow aspiration, in which 155 cases (52.2%) showed moderate proliferation. The remaining cases were normal.

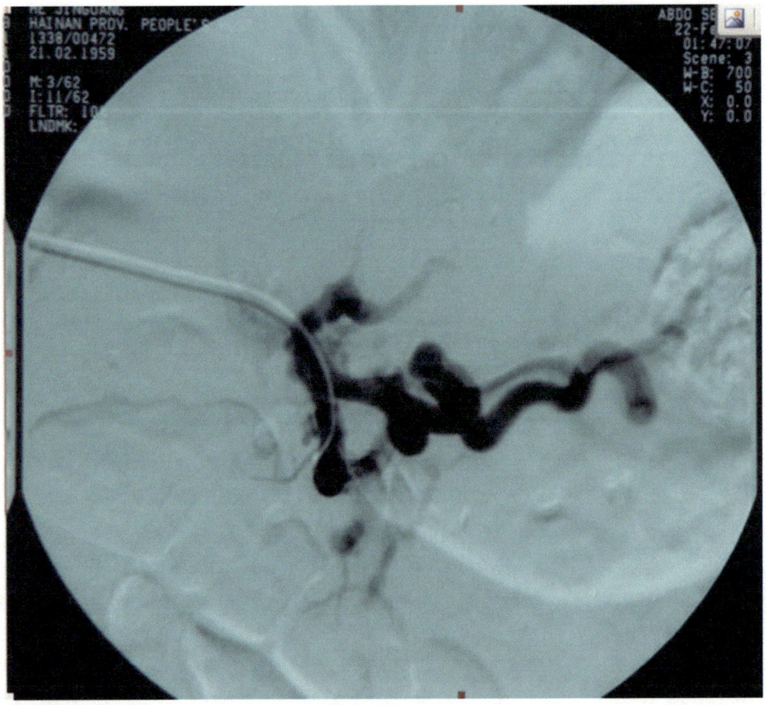

Fig. 1. severe varices in the distal esophagus and gastric fundus.

Item	N	%	WBC (×10⁹/L)	RBC (×10¹²/L)	PLT (×10⁹/L)
Pancytopenia	113	34.2	2.35±0.76 (median 2.36)	2.99±0.64 (median 3.00)	58.6±19.8 (median 57.8)
WBC+PLT	30	9.1	2.76±0.71 (median 2.73)	----	56.9±21.2 (median 53.8)
RBC+PLT	48	14.5	----	2.83±0.20 (median2.63)	67.2±21.3 (median 62.5)
WBC+RBC	40	12.1	2.85±0.76 (median 2.68)	3.11±0.30 (median 2.96)	-----
PLT	27	8.2	----	----	66.2±23.3 (median 61.7)
WBC	14	4.2	2.98±0.65 (median 2.82)	-----	-----
RBC	58	17.6	----	2.71±0.50 (median 2.56)	----

Note: The difference in WBC was significant between Group 1 and Group 2, 4 and 6 ($P<0.05$), and not significant between Group 2 and Group 4 and 6 ($P>0.05$); The difference in RBC was significant between Group 1 and Group 7, between Group 3 and Group 4, and between Group 4 and Group 7 ($P<0.05$), not significant between Group 1 and Group 3 and 4 ($P>0.05$), and not significant between Group 3 and Group 7 ($P>0.05$); And the difference in PLT was not significant when the 4 groups were compared ($P>0.05$, $F=1.61$).

Table 1. Hemocyte decrease (mean±SEM) in 330 cases ($\bar{x}$ ±s)

3. Causes of hemocytopenia in peripheral blood

There are numerous causes for cytopenias in patients with hepatocirrhotic portal hypertension, including the toxic effects of hepatic viruses and alcohol on the bone marrow, hypofunctioning of the liver [2], splenomegaly, hypersplenism, gastrointestinal bleeding, and hematopoietic dysfunction caused by malnutrition. In most cases, cytopenias are caused by multiple factors.

3.1 Toxic effects of hepatic virus

Hepatic viruses can directly suppress the differentiation and proliferation of hemopoietic stem cells and progenitor cells [3]. (2) Hepatic virus can cause disorders of cellular immunity and humoral immunity in vivo, to compromise the body's capacity to eliminate the viruses. The constant presence of viruses damages the hemopoietic functioning of the bone marrow [4]. (3) Viruses can impair the activity of bone marrow stromal cells to reduce the secretion of cytokines and to affect the proliferation of hemopoietic cells. (4) During pathogenesis caused by cytokines, the increase in the γ- interferon level and decrease in the interleukin-6 and erythropoietin levels, can affect the proliferation of hemopoietic cells [5]. The hepatitis B virus (HBV) and hepatitis C virus (HCV) can suppress the bone marrow, and affect the growth of all karyocytes in the bone marrow. This may lead to hypoplastic anemia, and patients must undergo a bone marrow transplant to survive.

The liver and bone marrow are target tissues of HBV. This virus can kill or injure hemopoietic cells directly, causing myelosuppression, and leading to leukopenia and reduction in the detoxification ability of the liver. This renders the body more sensitive to certain medicines, toxins and environmental pollutants, and cause hypofunctioning of bone marrow hematopoiesis. Leukopenia further damages immunity to cause the active replication of HBV, forming a vicious cycle. Currently, antiviral therapy is the first choice for chronic hepatitis B patients; however, antiviral medications also lead to myelosuppression. Therefore, monitoring leukocytes in the peripheral blood is conducive to the regulation of antiviral therapy. If the leukocyte count is lower than $2\times10^9/L$, antiviral therapy should be discontinued. Both HBV and HCV can induce suppression of the precursor cells of the bone marrow, and affect the lymph cells, causing lymphopenia and hypofunctioning of the bone marrow.

3.2 Toxic effects of alcohol

In the 1980s, studies of patients with alcoholic liver disease reported that neutrophil granulocytes demonstrated retarded growth and delayed release in the bone marrow. Later studies showed increased apoptosis of neutrophil granulocytes. Patients with end-stage cirrhosis complicated with neutropenia underwent Granulocyte-Macrophage Colony Stimulating Factor (GM-CSF) therapy for 7 days, and the leukocyte count increased more than 100%. However, the increased leukocytes could not be destroyed in the spleen, for no leukocyte fragments were found in the spleen. Ethanol can suppress or stimulate cellular proliferation, but in most cases, it suppresses cellular growth and increases cytotoxic effects. Its mechanism includes retarded cellular proliferation and induced apoptosis and necrosis [6-8]. A foreign study reported [9] that long-term alcoholism could cause abnormalities in the bone marrow and peripheral blood. In that study, 91% patients manifested changes in the peripheral blood including granulopenia, thrombopenia, etc., and changes in bone marrow included highly-differentiated hemopoietic tissue and myelofibrosis. Long-term alcohol consumption can reduce the absorption of folic acid and vitamin B_{12}, which impairs the synthesis of erythrocytes. Djordjevic et al [10] believed both that hepatic viruses and alcoholism were able to cause cytopenias.

3.3 Hypofunctioning of liver

Hypofunctioning of the liver reduces degradation of toxic metabolites by liver cells; in this case, the liver cannot detoxify the toxins that suppress the bone marrow, thus affecting hemopoietic function. The incidence of liver disease combined with thrombopenia is 15% - 70%. It is usually at mild or moderate level, and its severity is a prognostic indicator. In liver diseases, thrombopenia is closely related to hepatocirrhosis, anti-platelet autoantibodies [11], bone marrow suppression caused by HBV and HCV, and toxic effects from excessive alcohol consumption [12]. The discovery of thrombopoietin (TPO) in 1994 ushered in a new era in the study of cirrhotic thrombopenia. TPO is almost exclusively produced in liver cells; a small proportion of TPO is produced in the kidneys, bone marrow stromal cells and muscle. The production of TPO depends on the function and amount of liver cells. In cirrhosis, functional liver cells become less able to decrease the secretion of TPO. A study by Wolber et al. [13], of cirrhotic patients developing from the compensation to decompensation stage, demonstrated that the expression or serum level of TPO changed from an increase to a decrease, and that the platelet count decreased gradually. The decrease in liver function, to some extent, was related to hemocytopenia and bone marrow dysfunction. Forbes et al. [14] suggested that hepatic exogenous myofibroblasts played an important role in hepatic fibrosis. In hepatic fibrosis, bone marrow stem cells differentiate into hepatic endothelial parenchymal cells but not into myofibroblasts. This indicates that the change in hemopoietic function and inner environment of the bone marrow might be somehow related to or interactive with the occurrence and development of hepatic fibrosis or even hepatic cirrhosis. These observations suggest that changes in the bone marrow of cirrhotic patients do not result from one single factor but a combination of multiple factors, with a complicated regulation mechanism. The changes in bone marrow might be directly or indirectly related to the severity of hepatic cirrhosis and changes in liver or spleen function. Their relationship and the detailed mechanism remain to be further explored. Solving this puzzle will be of significant importance to clinical practice.

3.4 Splenomegaly and hypersplenism

Hypersplenism is secondary to splenomegaly. Two mechanisms for splenomegaly caused by liver diseases exist. The first mechanism is expansionary splenomegaly, including congestive splenomegaly caused by increased venous pressure and hyperemic splenomegaly caused by increased splenic arterial flow; the former is the main cause. The second mechanism is hypertrophic splenomegaly, including: (1) Hepatic virus antigen and exogenous antigens unprocessed by the liver due to a shunting procedure, can stimulate the spleen and lead to hypertrophy of the immune tissue in the spleen (splenic corpuscle, periarterial lymphatic sheath, marginal zone). (2) In hepatic cirrhosis, increased necrotic cells and hypofunctioning of the hepatic reticuloendothelial system promote compensatory hypertrophy and lead to hyperfunctioning of the splenic reticuloendothelial system. (3) Increased intrasplenic pressure, stasis of blood circulation, change in the metabolic environment and other factors can cause fibroplastic proliferation. Generally speaking, intrasplenic immune tissues show obvious hypertrophy during hepatitis, and middle or end stage cirrhotic patients mainly manifest splenic sinus dilation, hypertrophy of reticuloendothelial system and fibrous tissues.

Currently, there are several hypotheses concerning the mechanism of cytopenia: (1) The hypothesis of intrasplenic trapping[15]: After the formation of splenomegaly, blood volume in the spleen increases, and a great number of leukocytes, erythrocytes and platelets are trapped in the spleen. The ratio of trapped hemocytes compared with that in the normal spleen is 5.5- to 20-fold, resulting in hemocytopenia in the peripheral blood. (2) The hypothesis of cytophagy: There are a large number of mononuclear-macrophages in the spleen. Under pathological circumstances, mononuclear-macrophages demonstrate hyperfunctioning in cytophagy and destruction of hemocytes, especially erythrocytes [16]. Recently, a study using erythrocyte creatine (EC), the life-span sensitive marker of erythrocytes, revealed that the EC level was significantly increased in patients with splenomegaly due to post-necrotic cirrhosis compared with patients with hepatic cirrhosis with normal spleens ($P<0.05$). In addition, the same was observed compared with the normal control group but without a significant difference [17]. This suggested that splenomegaly accelerated the destruction of erythrocytes and the determination of the EC value could be used to evaluate the severity of cirrhotic splenomegaly [18]. (3) The spleen can produce excessive "splenic hormones" to suppress the hemopoietic function of the bone marrow, and accelerate the destruction of and trap produced hemocytes to prevent them from entering into blood circulation [19]. (4) The hypothesis of autoimmunity: The spleen is a large lymph organ that produces antibodies. Antigens unprocessed by the liver enter the marginal zones of splenic lymph follicles (splenic nodule) and activate the pro-lymphocytes and plasma cells to generate antibodies. These antibodies can destroy hemocytes causing hemocytopenia in the peripheral blood.

3.5 Gastrointestinal bleeding

Gastroesophageal fundus varices bleeding is a common complication for patients with cirrhotic portal hypertension. Gastrointestinal bleeding of any cause can directly lead to a decreased amount of hemocytes in the effective circulatory blood volume.

Chronic gastrointestinal bleeding can result in iron, folic acid and vitamin B_{12} deficiencies, and insufficient material for the synthesis of erythrocytes. Massive loss of erythrocytes can lead to anemia in patients. A Cr^{51} labeled-erythrocyte test demonstrated that only 20% of patients with cirrhosis complicated with anemia had increased erythrocytes in their spleens.

3.6 Malnutrition

Portal hypertensive gastropathy can cause malabsorption of hematopoietic growth factors and non-visible loss of nutrients necessary for hematopoiesis. Additionally, the lack of iron, folic acid and vitamin B_{12} results in insufficient materials for the synthesis of erythrocytes, leading to decreased hematopoiesis.

The significance of exploring the causes of hemocytopenia in the peripheral blood in the patients with cirrhotic portal hypertension lies in its guidance for treatment and evaluation for therapeutic effects. If hemocytopenia is caused by splenomegaly or hypersplenism, whether monolineage or multi-lineage, the decreased hemocytes will rise significantly after a splenectomy ($P<0.01$). The most sensitive is hemocyte is the platelet, which will increase half an hour after the operation, and reach the highest level in 2 weeks; afterwards it will decrease gradually and remain at a normal level. Leukocytes and erythrocytes would increase following the platelets. Hemocytopenia in the peripheral blood caused by non-splenic factors does not lead to a definite increase in hemocytes after splenectomy.

4. Hemocytopenia in peripheral blood and its prognosis

The postoperative prognosis was classified as cured, improved or dead. There were few cases without any changes. In this analysis, cured meant meeting the following criteria: the disappearance of ascites, abdominal distension and hemorrhage, blood cell count increase and recovery, improvement in liver function, no severe postoperative complications, and meeting the criteria for being discharged from the hospital. On the other hand, dead meant that the patients died during hospitalization, or that the patients in critical condition died one week after early discharge from the hospital, as requested by the relatives. All others were considered improved. Comparison of the therapeutic effect between each mono-lineage cytopenia group is shown in Table 2. Comparison of the therapeutic effect between mono-lineage cytopenia and bi-lineage and comparisons of the therapeutic effect between the mono-lineage cytopenia and bi-lineage cytopenias, the mono-lineage cytopenia and multi-lineage cytopenias are shown in Table3 and Table 4, respectively.

Group	Grade	Case number	Therapeutic effect			$\chi2$, P value
			Cured (%)	Improved (%)	Dead (%)	
WBC ($\times 10^9$/L, N=14)	<2	1	1 (100)	0	0	$\chi2$=1.478, P=0.478
	2-3	10	6(60)	4 (40)	0	
	3-4	3	1 (33.3)	2 (66.7)	0	
RBC ($\times 10^{12}$/L, N=58)	<2	4	3 (75)	0	1 (25)	$\chi2$=10.908 P=0.028<0.05
	2-3	20	16 (80)	2 (10)	2 (10)	
	3-4	34	16 (47.1)	16(47.1)	2 (5.8)	
PLT ($\times 10^9$/L, N=27)	<30	3	1 (33.3)	2 (66.7)	0	$\chi2$=2.220, P=0.695
	30-50	1	1 (100)	0	0	
	50-100	23	15 (65.2)	7 (30.4)	1 (4.4)	
HB (hemoglobin) ($\times$g/L, N=366)	<30	78	32 (41)	39 (50)	7(9)	$\chi2$=4.236, P=0.375
	30-70	52	28 (53.8)	20 (38.5)	4 (7.7)	
	>70	236	122 (51.7)	89 (37.7)	25 (10.6)	

Note: Among the four mono-lineage peripheral cytopenia groups, only the RBC group demonstrated a significant difference in intra-group comparison ($p<0.05$); comparison among the four groups revealed no significant difference ($P>0.05$).

Table 2. Comparison of the therapeutic effect between each mono-lineage peripheral cytopenia group

Table 2 shows that only the RBC group demonstrated a significant difference ($P<0.05$) in the intra-group comparison among the mono-lineage cytopenia groups. According to Table 3 and Table4, there were significant differences ($P<0.05$) in the therapeutic effects between mono-lineage cytopenias and multi-lineage cytopenias, indicating that the more severe the cytopenia, the worse the therapeutic results appeared to be.

For the multi-lineage cytopenias(Table5), a multiple linear regression analysis was applied, and results revealed that thrombocytopenia was the major factor ($P<0.005$) influencing the therapeutic effect, while leukopenia, erythropenia and decreased hemoglobin showed no statistical significance, and should not be considered. Erythropenia showed significant differences in the intra-group comparison of mono-lineage cytopenias, but no difference compared to other mono-lineage cytopenia groups. This was possibly due to the small sample size in the mono-lineage cytopenia groups. Leukopenia showed no significant difference in the univariate analysis or the multivariate analysis, and had no influence on the therapeutic results. For example, 2 patients recovered and were discharged from the hospital though their leukocyte count was lower than $1\times10^9/L$; this may have been because they had no serious postoperative infection. Theoretically, anemia is related to the prognosis, but in this research it showed no statistical significance in the univariate analysis or the multivariate analysis; the reason for this may have been because the blood transfusions before and during operation had a favorable effect on the blood condition. Although thrombocytopenia had no statistical significance in the univariate analysis, in the multiple linear regression analysis it was indicated to be the most important influential factor with the increase in case load.

Item	Total case number	Therapeutic effect			$\chi2$, P value
		Cured (%)	Improved (%)	Dead (%)	
Mono-lineage cytopenia	99	60 (60.6%)	33 (33.3%)	6 (6.1%)	$\chi2$=7.446, P=0.024
Bi-lineage cytopenia	118	51 (43.2%)	51 (43.2%)	16 (13.6%)	

Table 3. Comparison of the therapeutic effect between the mono-lineage cytopenia and bi-lineage cytopenia

Item	Total case number	Therapeutic effect			$\chi2$, P value
		Cured (%)	Improved (%)	Dead (%)	
Mono-lineage cytopenia	99	60 (60.6)	33 (33.3)	6 (6.1)	$\chi2$=7.819, P=0.02
Multi-lineage cytopenia	231	102 (44.2)	102 (44.2)	27 (11.6)	

Table 4. Comparison of the therapeutic effect between the mono-lineage cytopenia and tri-lineage cytopenia

Thrombocytopenia is a significant and common complication in posthepatitic cirrhotic portal hypertension[20-21]; it is related to not only retention of blood cell in the spleen, blood cell aggregation and enhanced phagocytosis of macrophages[22], but also HBV infection, and compensation and regulation of marrow[23]. Djordevic et al[10]. proposed that extreme thrombocytopenia was life-threatening. A PLT count of < $30x10^9/L$ can cause variceal hemorrhaging in the distal esophagus and gastric fundus, and intraoperative and postoperative massive wound hemorrhaging, which can be life-threatening. Therefore, PLT transfusions should be performed before an operation to increase the PLT count to $50\times10^9/L$ to ensure the safety of the patient. Cui et al[24]. reported that PLT transfusions combined with plasma fibrinogen transfusions led to better results. In some cases, after transfusion of 12-24 units of PLT, the PLT count did not increase obviously, or decreased to the previous lowest count after 1-2 days. These types of patients are suitable for splenectomy[25]. Mastuura et al.[26]suggested that the excessive postoperative PLT count was also a life-threatening factor, so the condition of the patient should be closely monitored[27-28] when there is excessive platelet count, appropriate treatment should be administrated immediately.

Item	T value	*P* value
PLT	2.827	.005
RBC	-.439	.661
WBC	1.516	.130
HB	0.628	0.531
Constant	1.395	.000

Note: Regression equation $\hat{Y}$ =1.395+0.151 PLT

Table 5. Multiple linear regression analysis of blood cells in 366 cases

5. Grading of hemocytopenia

In 1907, Chauffard proposed the term 'hypersplenism' for the first time[29]. After further research, in 1949, Doan[30] proposed the criteria for hypersplenism: 1. enlarged spleen 2. mono-lineage or multi-lineage cytopenias 3. normal or proliferative bone marrow 4. disappearance of the pathological changes in the blood components after splenectomy. While these four criteria are indispensable for the diagnosis of hypersplenism, peripheral cytopenia and an increase and recovery in blood cell count after a splenectomy are the major criteria for assessing hypersplenism due to cirrhotic portal hypertension. This is because splenomegaly in itself is a necessary criterion for the cirrhotic portal hypertension.

It is of vital significance to formulate a grading method, like the Child-Pugh Classification for liver function, to evaluate hypersplenism. However, grading of hypersplenism is extremely difficult for many reasons. 1) Some patients show decreased monolineage cytopenias and others show bi-lineage cytopenias. Even patients with pancytopenia barely meet the grading criteria. 2) There are many causes of hemocytopenia, but no examination can ascertain whether it is caused by splenomegaly or hypersplenism. A definite diagnosis would be made only when hemocytes returned to a normal level after splenectomy.

Although grading of hypersplenism is difficult, hemocytopenia could be graded. According to a multiple linear regression, thrombopenia is the major factor influencing the effect of surgery. The 330 cases of cytopenia scores were mainly based on thrombocytopenia combined with erythropenia, as well as clinical experience (leukopenia). Scoring was as follows: PLT>$50<100x10^9/L$ was scored as 1 point, $30\text{-}50x10^9/L$ was scored as 2 points, $<30x10^9/L$ was scored as 3 points; RBC $3\text{-}4x10^{12}/L$ was scored as 0 points, and RBC$<3x10^{12}/L$ was scored as 1 point; WBC $2\text{-}4x10^9/L$ was scored as 0 points, and

WBC<2x10^9/L was scored as 1 point. Except for 36 cases with normal blood cell counts and 69 cases with 0 points, the influences of scores on postoperative prognoses in 261 cases are shown in Table 6 (totally 105 cases). There were significant differences between the 3 groups ($P<0.05$). Therefore, peripheral cytopenias were graded as mild (<2), medium (2-3) or severe (>3) (Table 7).

Thus, only cytopenias can be graded. In the present study, the cases were scored and graded based on the accumulated scores. The scoring criteria used in this study were: 1.Analytical results of multiple linear regression: F value obtained from multiple linear regression equation was 7.993 ($P<0.005$), indicating that multiple linear regression was applicable. The equation $\hat{Y}$=1.395+0.151PLT indicated that thrombocytopenia was the major influential factor for postoperative prognosis. Therefore, according to the severity of the thrombocytopenia, 1 to 3 points was scored. 2. Intra-group comparison of erythropenia showed a significant difference ($P<0.05$), so an RBC count ≤3x10^{12}/L was scored as 1 point. 3. According to clinical experience, leukopenia can cause severe infection and lead to undesirable effects. A WBC of count ≤2x10^9/L was scored as 1 point, though leukopenia showed no statistical significance in either the univariate analysis or multivariate analysis. A total score of <2 points indicated mild cytopenia, 2-3 points indicated medium cytopenia and >3 points indicated severe cytopenia. If cytopenias are caused by hypersplenism, this grading standard could also be used for grading hypersplenism or as a reference.

Item	Total case number	Therapeutic effect			χ2, P value
		Cured (%)	Improved (%)	Death (%)	
1 point	136	80 (58.8%)	43(31.6%)	13 (9.6%)	
2-3 points	95	41 (43.2%)	44 (46.3%)	10 (10.5%)	χ2=10.163 P=0.034
4-5 points	30	10 (33.3%)	15 (50%)	5 (16.7%)	

Table 6. Comparison of the influence of different scores on the therapeutic effect

Item	Mild	Medium	Severe
PLT	>50	30-50	<30
(Score)	1	2	3
RBC	>3	2-3	<2
(Score)	0	1	1
WBC	>3	2-3	<2
(Score)	0	0	1
Total score	<2	2-3	>3

Table 7. Grading of peripheral cytopenias (hypersplenism)

Cytopenia grading could facilitate clinical practice in various aspects, including assessing the disease condition, representation and academic communication, communication with patients and their relatives to resolve or avoid medical disputes, choosing a suitable treatment plan (for example, splenectomy is suitable for severe cytopenia or hypersplenism) and taking preventive methods before an operation[16] to increase the curative rate.

6. Treatment

As to the patients with splenomegaly due to cirrhotic portal hypertension complicated with hemocytopenia in the peripheral blood, treatment should aim at both the causes and clinical symptoms, that is, the principle of treating the branch and the root simultaneously.

6.1 Treatment of causes of disease

- Antiviral treatment: Patients with severe viral infection should take antiviral medicine for an extended time, and should be constantly monitored to protect liver function.
- Avoid drinking alcohol: Patients with alcoholic cirrhosis and post-hepatic cirrhosis should avoid drinking alcohol; otherwise, disease conditions may deteriorate. In addition, medications that affect liver function should be avoided.
- Correcting malnutrition: Patients with obvious emaciation and malabsorption should replenish nutrients, such as iron, folic acid and vitamin B_{12} to avoid a shortage of materials for the synthesis of erythrocytes. Additionally, patients should undergo blood transfusions to treat anemia and increase the hemochrome level.

6.2 Treatment of symptoms

Different treatments should be applied according to the severity of the disease. Patients with mild hemocytopenia should be under close observation; for patients with moderate hemocytopenia, blood components or whole blood transfusions should be applied as well as hemocyte boosting medications. In severe cases, a splenectomy in the patients with splenomegaly should be considered. Theoretically, splenic arterial embolization can also achieve the same effect as a splenectomy, but this procedure tends to cause splenic infarction, splenic necrosis, splenic abscess and high fever. This method should only be attempted by experienced physicians.

In recent years, autologous stem cell transplantation has achieved good results in the treatment of cirrhotic portal hypertension complicated with hemocytopenia in the peripheral blood [17], but more research is needed to further its application in clinics.

6.3 Treatment of both the branch and root: Treating the causes and the clinical symptoms

1. Gastrointestinal bleeding: Gastrointestinal bleeding is not only a cause of hemocytopenia in peripheral blood, but also a complication of cytopenia. It is of vital importance to treat gastrointestinal bleeding; treatment measures include blood transfusion, fluid infusion, intravenous injection of antacid, administration of somatostatin (sandostatin and stilamin), endoscopic loop ligation of bleeding areas, sclerotherapy, and so on. Lecleire et al. [31] demonstrated that the success rate of endoscopic treatment could reach 80%. Intervention embolization can also be applied. Selective embolization can stop the bleeding in most cases. In recent years, with the improvement of coaxial catheter and embolization material, super-selective angiography and transcatheter embolization (SATE) is regarded as a safe and effective method to treat gastrointestinal hemorrhage[32]. It should be the first choice for patients suffering from post-operational massive hemorrhage, especially for the elderly or the sick. If the intervention fails, surgery should be performed.

If massive hemorrhage cannot be stopped using the measures mentioned above, emergency surgery should be performed, including pericardial devascularization and/or placement of a transjugular intrahepatic portal systemic shunt.

2. Liver transplantation: Schuppan et al. [33] concluded that liver transplantation was an effective method to treat cirrhotic portal hypertension, as it not only corrected liver problems, but also cured portal hypertension, and was likely an effective way to treat hemocytopenia. After transplantation, the TPO level increases immediately. In 2 or 3 days, the TPO level can be 5-10 times the level it was before the surgery. In about 6 days, the platelet count returns to the normal range, and anemia is corrected. Therefore, liver transplantation can treat both the branch and root simultaneously.

7. References

[1] Wu ZD, Wu ZH. Surgery. 7th Edition[M]. People's Medical Publishing House, 2008, 525-532.

[2] Bashour FN, Teran JC, Mullen KD. Prevalence of peripheral blood cytopenias (hypersplenism) in patients with nonalcoholic chronic liver disease[J]. Gastroenterology,2000,95 (10): 2936-2939.

[3] Van E, Niele AM, Kroes AC. Human parvovirus B19: relevance in internal medicine[J]. Neth J Med, 1999, 54(6):221-230.

[4] Kevin E.Brown, John Tisdale, A John Barrett, et al. Hepatitis-associated aplastic anemia[J]. N Engl J Med, 1997, 336:1059-1064.

[5] Dilloo D, Vohringer R, Josting A, et al. Bone marrow fibroblasts from children with aplastic anemia exhibit reduced interlukin-6 production in response to cytokines and viral challenge[J]. Pediatr Res, 1995, 38(5):716-721.

[6] Young NS, Maciejewski J. The pathophysiology of acquired aplastic anemia[J]. N Engl J Med,1997,336(19):1365-1372.

[7] Jacobs JS, Miller MW. Proliferation and deat h of cultured fetal neocortical neurons:effects of ethanol on the dynamics of cell growth[J]. J Neurocytol, 2001,30 (5):391-401.

[8] Hao LP, Hu XF, Pang H, et al. The study on apoptosis and its molecular mechanism in mouse insulinama cells induced by ethanol[J]. J Toxicol, 2006, 20(3):138-140.

[9] Neuman MG, Haber JA, Malkiewicz IM, et al. Ethanol signals for apoptosis in cultured skin cells[J]. Alcohol, 2002, 26(3):179-190.

[10] Djordjević J, Svorcan P, Vrinić D, Dapcević B.Splenomegaly and thrombocytopenia in patients with liver cirrhosis. Vojnosanit Pregl.2010 Feb: 67(2):166-9.

[11] Sezai S, Kamisaka K, Ikegami F, et al. Regulation of hepatic thrombopoietin production by portal hemodynamics in liver cirrhosis[J]. Am J Gastroenterol, 1998, 93(1):80-82.

[12] Lu-Yunfu,Yue Jie, Gong Xiaoguang,, et al. Anaemia of Cirrhotic Portal Hypertension with Hypersplenism.Journal of Surgery:Concepts & Practice, 2009, 14 (6): 669-670.

[13] Wolber EM, Ganschow R, Burdelski M, et al. Hepatic thrombopoietin mRNA levels in acute and chronic liver failure of childhood[J]. Hepatology, 1999, 29(6):1739-1742.

[14] Forbes SJ, Russo FP, Rey V, et al. A significant proportion of myofibroblasts are of bone marrow origin in human liver fibrosis[J].Gastroenterology,2004,126(4): 955-963.

[15] Shah SH, Hayes PC, Allan PL,et al. Measurement of spleen size and its relation to hypersplenism and portal hemodynamics in portal hypertension due to hepatic cirrhosis[J]. Am J Gastroenterol,1996,91(12):2580-2583

[16] Jiao YF, Okumiya T, Saibara T, et al. Erythrocyte creatine as a marker of excessive erythrocyte destruction due to hypersplenism in patients with liver cirrhosis[J]. Clin Biochem, 2001, 34(5):395-398.
[17] Friedman LS. The risk of surgery in patients with liver disease. Hepatology, 1999, 29:1617-1623.
[18] Zhou Yongxing. Modern Diagnostics & Therapeutics of Liver Cirrhosis. 1st edition. Beijing: People's Military Medical Press, 2002: 247-249.
[19] Faeh M, Hauser SP, Nydegger UE. Transient thrombopoietin peak after liver transplantation for end-stage liver disease[J]. Br J Haematol, 2001, 112(2):493- 498.
[20] Karasu Z, Gurakar A, Kerwin B,et al. Effect of transjuqular intrahepatic portosystemic shunt on thrombocytopenia associated with cirrhosis. Dig Dis Sci,2001Feb, 46 (2): 449-456.
[21] Fadi NB, J Carlos T, Kevin D, et al.Prevalence of Peripheral Blood Cytopenias (Hypersplenism) in Patients With Nonalcoholic Liver Disease. Am Coll of Gastroeterology, 2000, 95(10): 2937-2939.
[22] Yan F, Li W, Gao J, et al. cDN Amicoarray--based screening of differentially expressed genes in macrophages in the spleen of patients with portal Hypertension and hypersplenism. Nan Fang Yi Ke Da Xue Xue Bao 2006;26(11):1548-1551.
[23] Yun-fu L, Xin-qiu L, Xian-he X, et al. Portal Hypertension Splenomegaly is not Always Associated with Hematocytopenia. J of US-China Medical Science, 2009,6 (1):28-30.
[24] Cui Y, Hei F, Long C, Feng Z,et al. Perioperative monitoring of thromboelastograph on hemostasis and therapy for cyanotic infants undergoing complex cardiac surgery. Artif Organs.2009 Nov; 33(11):909-14.
[25] Li-xinqiao,Lu-yunfu, Huang wei-wei, *et al.*Peripheral Blood Cell Variety in Patients with Hypersplenism Secondary to Hepatic Cirrhosis accompanied with Portal Hypertension. Chinese Journal Of General Surgery,2007, 22 (9): 702.
[26] Matsuura T, Hayashida M, Saeki I, Taguchi T.The risk factors of persistent thrombocytopenia and splenomegaly after liver transplantation.Pediatr Surg Int.2010 Oct;26(10):1007-10.
[27] Johansson PI, Stensballe J.Hemostatic resuscitation for massive bleeding: the paradigm of plasma and platelets--a review of the current literature. Transfusion. 2010 Mar;50(3):701-10. Epub 2009 Nov 19.
[28] Shontz R, Karuparthy V, Temple R,et al.Prevalence and risk factors predisposing to coagulopathy in patients receiving epidural analgesia for hepatic surgery. Reg Anesth Pain Med.2009 Jul-Aug;34(4):308-11.
[29] Fadi NB, J Carlos T, Kevin D, et al.Prevalence of Peripheral Blood Cytopenias (Hypersplenism) in Patients With Nonalcoholic Liver Disease. Am Coll of Gastroeterology, 2000, 95 (10): 2937-2939.
[30] Doan CA.Hypersplenism. Bull N Y Acad Med. 1949 Oct;25(10):625-50.
[31] Lecleire S, Ben-Soussan E, Antonietti M, et al.Bleeding gastric vascular treated by argon plasma coagulation: a comparison between patients with and without cirrhosis. Gastrointes Endosc,2008,67 (2): 219-225.
[32] Fishman SJ, Shamberger RC, Fox VL, Burrows PE, Endorectal pull-through abates gastrointestinal hemorrhage from colorectal venous malformations. J Pediatr Surg. 2000 Jun;35(6):982-4.
[33] Schuppan D,Afdha NH. Liver cirrhosis. Lancet,2008,371 (9615): 838-851.